Genders and Sexualities in History

Palgrave Macmillan's series, Genders and Sexualities in History, accommodates and fosters new approaches to historical research in the fields of genders and sexualities. The series promotes world-class scholarship, which concentrates upon the interconnected themes of genders, sexualities, religions/religiosity, civil society, politics and war.

Historical studies of gender and sexuality have, until recently, been more or less disconnected fields. In recent years, historical analyses of genders and sexualities have synthesised, creating new departures in historiography. The additional connectedness of genders and sexualities with questions of religion, religiosity, development of civil societies, politics and the contexts of war and conflict is reflective of the movements in scholarship away from narrow history of science and scientific thought, and history of legal processes approaches, that have dominated these paradigms until recently. The series brings together scholarship from Contemporary, Modern, Early Modern, Medieval, Classical and Non-Western History. The series provides a diachronic forum for scholarship that incorporates new approaches to genders and sexualities in history.

Douglas Pretsell

Queer Voices in the Works of Richard von Krafft-Ebing, 1883–1901

palgrave
macmillan

Douglas Pretsell
La Trobe University
Melbourne, VIC, Australia

ISSN 2730-9479 ISSN 2730-9487 (electronic)
Genders and Sexualities in History
ISBN 978-3-031-17330-1 ISBN 978-3-031-17331-8 (eBook)
https://doi.org/10.1007/978-3-031-17331-8

Cover illustration: History and Art Collection / Alamy Stock Photo

This Palgrave Macmillan imprint is published by the registered company Springer Nature Switzerland AG.
The registered company address is: Gewerbestrasse 11, 6330 Cham, Switzerland

Series Editor Preface

Douglas Pretsell's superb book *Queer Voices in the Works of Richard von Krafft-Ebing, 1883–1901* is a genuinely ground-breaking critical source edition of the 'case studies' of late nineteenth-century Queer people who submitted autobiographical accounts of their sexuality to the foundational sexologist, Richard von Krafft-Ebing. In this highly original, timely and invaluable critical source edition, Pretsell provides new translations for the first time in English from the original German and brings to the fore Queer 'case studies' seen in Krafft-Ebing's *Psychopathia Sexualis*, first published in Germany in 1886 and thereafter in repeated editions. *Psychopathia Sexualis* was an original text in sexology with global significance in the categorisation of sex and sexualities. Queer people corresponded with Krafft-Ebing often to contest and challenge the pathologisation and ubiquitous social opprobrium of same-sex desire and gender variance and this is reflected in many of the fascinating 'case studies' here. The 'case studies' often reinforced the authors' sexual identification, not dissimilar to LGBTQ+ 'coming out' stories today. In common with all volumes in the 'Genders and Sexualities in History' series, *Queer Voices in the Works of Richard von Krafft-Ebing, 1883–1901* is a multifaceted and meticulously researched scholarly study and is a sophisticated contribution to our understanding of the past.

London, UK — Joanna Bourke
London, UK — Sean Brady
Melbourne, VIC, Australia — Matthew Champion

Acknowledgements

This book is a companion to my other critical edition, *The Correspondence of Karl Heinrich Ulrichs, 1846–1894*. Both these critical editions profile two constellations of primary sources that I am using in my forthcoming book on the men who called themselves 'urnings' in late nineteenth century Germany.

It has been a pleasure once again to work with Michael-Lombardi Nash. Michael is the translator of all of Karl Heinrich Ulrichs's works and some of the works of Magnus Hirschfeld. He has been a mentor to me as I embarked on the study of this period as well as my translator of choice to work with. Professor Steven Smith of Hofstra University translated each of the passages in Latin that Krafft-Ebing had used to obscure the more sexually frank parts of some of the case studies. I am hugely grateful to my friend and the copyeditor of this book, Camille Nurka. It is always a pleasure to work with her. I am also thankful to Emily Russell at Palgrave Macmillan for her professional management and support, Sean Brady for encouraging me to submit a proposal and the series editors for 'Genders and Sexualities in History' for approving the proposal.

Most of the primary research for this book—the sourcing and translation of texts—was conducted in the midst of the COVID-19 pandemic, with Melbourne the most locked-down city on earth. The International Loans team at La Trobe University Library was repeatedly able to track down obscure texts with utmost efficiency and courtesy. My colleagues in the Department of History at La Trobe have been supportive throughout and I am particularly thankful to my supervisor, Dr Tim Jones, for his advice and for reading through the final draft. Finally, my thanks go to my long-suffering husband, Peter, who has put up with all my late nights writing, translating and compiling this book.

Translator's Note

Douglas and I share a deep interest in the history of queer emancipation and sexology in late nineteenth-century Germany—Douglas as a historian and I as a translator of nineteenth-century German, in particular the works of Karl Heinrich Ulrichs. So it was a delight when he asked me to collaborate with him by translating the autobiographies in *Queer Voices in the Works of Richard von Krafft-Ebing, 1883–1901*. This is my second collaboration with Douglas. In 2020, I teamed up with him for the translation of Ulrichs's letters in another Palgrave book: *The Correspondence of Karl Heinrich Ulrichs, 1846–1894*.[1] Those letter translations and the translations of case studies in the present book give the English reader access to archives of substantial historical interest to those charting the early years of sexual modernity.

The collaboration in the present book was simple. Douglas transcribed the case studies and completed an initial electronic translation of each. He then supplied me by email with a split-page document rendering the original German on the left, and on the right, the computer-aided translation. The computer translation using deepl.com provided a good rough translation but not good enough to publish without my contribution in reworking the translations. Autobiography is perhaps the easiest literary form to translate, especially when written by persons from the non-professional public at large, where legal and medical matters are kept to a minimum. Some sections of the case studies included passages in Latin where Krafft-Ebing had judged the content to be too racy to publish. Professor Steven

Smith of Hofstra University aided in the translation of Krafft-Ebing's inexpert Latin. All in all, this translation collaboration with Douglas and Steven on this project proved to be simple and easy and a pleasure to be a part of.

I should also mention that this book and Douglas's earlier book of letter translations form part of a much larger publishing effort by a number of academics to catalogue, translate and critically examine the published and unpublished works by and related to Karl Heinrich Ulrichs in time to celebrate the 2025 bicentenary of Ulrichs's birth. In the last couple of years, this project has also involved the translation of Ulrichs's Latin works: *Apicula Latina* (*Little Latin Bee*),[2] *Fori reconventionis* (*On Cross-Litigation*)[3] and *Alaudae* (*The Larks*, Ulrichs's Latin newspaper)[4]. Douglas provided particularly helpful suggestions for classical translators to work with me on these. Finally, I should mention that Douglas's critical editions of Ulrichs's letters and this edition of Krafft-Ebing's case study autobiographies are also related to a forthcoming book of his, the manuscript of which I have read, on the men who called themselves 'urnings' in late nineteenth century Germany.[5] Once that book and my translated works are published, we will together have published the English translations of Ulrichs's entire known body of Latin and German work. No wonder I accepted his offer to collaborate.

Michael Lombardi-Nash

Notes

1. Douglas Pretsell, *The Correspondence of Karl Heinrich Ulrichs, 1846–1894* (Cham: Palgrave Macmillan, 2020).
2. Karl Heinrich Ulrichs, *Little Latin Bee (Book II): Translated Latin and German Student Songs Including the Original Latin and German Version*, trans. Mark Masterson and Michael Lombardi-Nash (Kindle, 2020).
3. Karl Heinrich Ulrichs, *On Cross-Litigation*, trans. Peter Dennistoun Bryant (Kindle, forthcoming).
4. Karl Heinrich Ulrichs, *The Larks, or Songbirds: Translated and Edited from the Original Latin of Karl Heinrich Ulrichs* (London: Bloomsbury, forthcoming).
5. This book is currently under consideration by an academic publisher and will hopefully be available in the coming year.

A Note on the Text

The original digital copies of the published case studies were extracted from various sources. The internet archive (https://archive.org/) was the source of most of the editions of *Psychopathia Sexualis* (volumes 1, 3, 4, 5, 9 and 10), the 1890 and 1891 copies of *Neue Forschungen auf dem Gebiet der Psychopathia Sexualis*, the 1901 edition of Hirschfeld's *Jahrbuch* containing Krafft-Ebing's last article on *Neue Forschungen*, the *Lehrbuch der Psychiatrie* from 1883 and Krafft-Ebing's 1885 article in *Jarbücher für Psychiatrie.* The second edition of *Psychopathia Sexualis* came from the Bibliothèque nationale de France, the sixth edition was supplied by interlibrary loan from Zentralbibliothek (ZB) Frankfurt/Main (Universitätsbibliothek JC Senckenberg), the seventh from the Wellcome Library, the eighth from Cornell Library and the eleventh edition from the University of British Columbia Library. I obtained Krafft-Ebing's 1864 article in *Friedrich's Blatter* from the website of the Die Bayerische Staatsbibliothek, the 1877 article in *Archiv für Psychiatrie und Nervenkrankheiten* from the HathiTrust Digital Library website and Krafft-Ebing's papers in *Allgemeine Zeitschrift für Psychiatrie* (1882), *Der Irrenfreund* (1886) and *Friedrich's Blatter* (1891) via subito e. V. document delivery, where the source was not identified.

The case studies were first translated electronically into English using www.deepl.com and then each translation was corrected and finessed by the veteran translator of Ulrichs and Hirschfeld, Dr Michael Lombardi-Nash. Latin passages were translated by Hofstra University Professor Steven Smith. In the book, the case studies have been sorted into nine groups (see Introduction) and numbered accordingly with the source of the original case study and each of its subsequent repetitions in successive volumes of *Psychopathia Sexualis* provided in the annotation. Each case study has a number within each group and it is these numbers that are used to identify specific case studies within the introduction (2.1, 3.6, 4.2 etc.). The 'queer voice' within each case study, the words of the man or woman themselves, is represented with plain text. Any paraphrasing of the subject's words or explanatory text from Krafft-Ebing is italicised and enclosed in square brackets. Translations from passages Krafft-Ebing rendered in Latin are also italicised in squared brackets. Finally, footnotes are used for any notes that were contained in the original published case studies with chapter endnotes for all explanatory references added by me.

Terminology

In the period under discussion, the terminology used in the German-speaking world for same-sex attracted individuals was in a state of transition. There were three words used in the psychiatric literature. First, there is the neologism 'urning', introduced by the campaigner Karl Heinrich Ulrichs, a term widely used by same-sex attracted men about themselves in this period.[1] This was soon joined by a clinical term, *conträre Geschlechtsempfindung* (contrary sexual feeling), invented in 1869 by the director of mental and nervous diseases at the Charité Hospital in Berlin, Karl Friedrich Otto Westphal.[2] In the initial editions of *Psychopathia Sexualis*, Krafft-Ebing used both the words 'urning' and his own version of Westphal's neologism 'contra-sexual' to describe same-sex attracted men and women. The first mention of the word 'homosexual' appeared in one of the 1887 autobiographies where a well-read twenty-seven-year-old wrote: 'By a happy coincidence—and I still praise those days today—I was introduced to Plato's *Symposium* and Jäger's homosexual idiosyncrasy at almost the same time' (5.3).[3] Krafft-Ebing started using the word 'homosexual' himself from the 1889 edition onwards.[4] The relative balance between his use of the words 'urning' and the increasing use of 'homosexual' from 1889 onwards gives a crude measure of the penetration of the new terminology.[5] In his final edited volume in 1901, Krafft-Ebing had stopped using the 'urning' terminology and only used 'homosexual'. Throughout his writings, Krafft-Ebing used contra-sexual as the overarching terminology, but the words urning and homosexual were used interchangeably as synonyms for same-sex attracted men. This mixed usage of terminology will be reflected in the foregoing discussion.

Notes

1. Ulrichs derived the term from Plato's Symposium as the source for his neologism: 'My terminology is derived from the names of the gods Uranus and Dione. A poetical piece of fiction by Plato traced the origins of man-manly love to Uranus, the love for women to Dione.' Karl Heinrich Ulrichs, *Vindex*. Leipzig: H. Matthes, 1865. Translated by Michael Lombardi-Nash as 'Book One: Vindex' in *The Riddle of 'Man-Manly' Love: The Pioneering Work on Male Homosexuality*, vol. 1 (Buffalo: Prometheus Books, 1994), §2, 34.
2. Carl Friedrich Otto Westphal, 'Die conträre Sexualempfindung: Symptom eines neuropathischen (psychopathischen) Zustandes', *Archiv für Psychiatrie und Nervenkrankheiten* 2 (1869): 92–94.
3. Richard von Krafft-Ebing, *Psychopathia Sexualis. Mit besonderer Berücksichtigung der conträren Sexualempfindung: Eine klinisch-forensische Studie*, 2nd ed. (Stuttgart: Ferdinand Enke, 1887), 88.
4. Curiously, in the 1889 edition, Krafft-Ebing did not discuss why he started using the new terminology. Richard von Krafft-Ebing, *Psychopathia Sexualis: Mit besonderer Berücksichtigung der conträren Sexualempfindung. Eine klinisch-forensische Studie*, 4th ed. (Stuttgart: Ferdinand Enke, 1889), 74 & ff.
5. In 1889, Krafft-Ebing still used 'urning' 79% of the time and 'homosexual' 21%. That proportion grew steadily in subsequent volumes and by 1898 he was using 'homosexual' 40% of the time.

Contents

About the Author

Douglas Pretsell is a researcher in the Department of History at La Trobe University, Melbourne, Australia. He recently completed a Doctorate in History with a thesis entitled 'The Age of the Urning: Queer Identities and Advocacy in Germany, 1864-1897'. Douglas is also the author of another Palgrave Critical Edition: *The Correspondence of Karl Heinrich Ulrichs, 1846–1894* (Cham: Palgrave Macmillan, 2020). With previous research experience in psychology and neuroscience, Douglas brings a fresh perspective to the study of sexual science in nineteenth-century Austria and Germany.

List of Tables

CHAPTER 1

Introduction

Richard von Krafft-Ebing's *Psychopathia Sexualis*, published in multiple editions from 1886, has been described as the foundational text in sexology. A globally important atlas of sexual categories, it was translated into Russian, Italian, Hungarian, Dutch, Japanese and English. Embedded within the text, alongside the clinically derived case studies, were the voices of multiple queer men and women who had written their own sexual autobiographies for Krafft-Ebing. These voices are contained within the forty-one autobiographical case studies collected, translated into English and collated in the present volume.

Many of the case studies presented here were written by people who had contacted the psychiatrist Krafft-Ebing offering intimate insights into the most secret corners of their lives so that they might contest the social, psychological and legal consequences of the culturally pervasive condemnation of their sexual natures. When these case studies were written, in Austria under Paragraph 129 all same-sex sexual activity by both men and women was punished with imprisonment.[1] In Germany, 'unnatural fornication' between men was proscribed by Paragraph 175.[2] Initially this applied only to proven cases of anal sex but the law's reach had been further extended following a ruling by the Reichsgericht (Supreme Court) in Leipzig in 1879 to cover all acts between men 'similar to sexual intercourse' hinging on 'thrusting movements' for that similarity, thus

D. Pretsell, *Queer Voices in the Works of Richard von Krafft-Ebing, 1883–1901*, Genders and Sexualities in History,
https://doi.org/10.1007/978-3-031-17331-8_1

incorporating oral and interfemoral sex.[3] Legal prohibition, social conservatism and widespread religious belief meant that a pall of repressive intolerance suffused the very existence of the men and women who revealed themselves in writing to Krafft-Ebing. They were doing so in defiance of society at large and a hostile medical establishment. While some of his patients were compelled by the authorities or families to seek help from Krafft-Ebing, most of the autobiographers wrote to him of their own volition, and the motivation to write came from a desire to have their own stories and perspectives inscribed within the psychiatric record.

Krafft-Ebing was not the first to use sexual autobiography in clinical publications; Johann Ludwig Casper had famously published a 'self-confession of a pederast' in 1863 and Friedrich Scholz included a self-penned confession of one of his patients in 1873.[4] However, in the works of Krafft-Ebing, the sexual autobiographies of same-sex attracted men, and to a lesser extent women, became a central and defining feature of his casuistic approach. In this sense, Krafft-Ebing's approach was entirely different from any of his contemporaries. This critical introduction to Krafft-Ebing's sexual autobiographies will survey the historical background to the emergence of autobiography in Krafft-Ebing's works before proceeding with a narrative guide for the reader to help navigate the nine categories of case study contained in this book.

1.1 Historical Background

Sex, Psychiatry and the Law

Richard von Krafft-Ebing was born in 1840 in Mannheim, a city located between the rivers Rhine and Neckar in the Grand Duchy of Baden. His family was semi-aristocratic, and he had several relatives in senior legal positions. His father was the Chief Magistrate of the Grand Duchy, and his mother was the daughter of Carl Joseph Anton Mittermaier, one of the leading progressive legal scholars of the nineteenth century. Krafft-Ebing studied medicine in various locations, graduating from the Ruprecht-Karls-University in Heidelberg in 1863. He was first exposed to a new focus in psychiatry that summer, when he attended lectures on the role of the brain in mental illness given by Wilhelm Griesinger at the Burghölzi hospital in Zurich.[5] Griesinger's research heralded a 'new psychiatry' where every mental illness or aberration would be localised in the brain:

> Psychiatry has undergone a transformation in its relation to the rest of medicine. ... This transformation rests principally on the realization that patients with so-called 'mental illnesses' are really individuals with illnesses of the nerves and brain.[6]

Griesinger and his colleagues at the Charité hospital were strongly influenced by the hereditary degeneration theories promulgated by Benedict Morel and expanded by Valentin Magnan. Mental disorders, and any deviation from the norm, were seen to be the result of some ancestral pollution or stimulation—an alcoholic parent, for example—that generated lapses and deviations in the next generation. In this way, facets of behaviour or personality that had attracted legal censure were now reclassified as brain diseases. It was this experience and the theories Griesinger promoted about his research that convinced the young Krafft-Ebing to pursue a career in psychiatry.

'New psychiatry' was research-based and brain-centred, and it would also extend to cover domains well beyond the psychiatric institution. In particular, the realm of expert witnesses in the court system was increasingly colonised by forensic psychiatrists, occluding and marginalising the forensic examiner. As a consequence, the examination of 'pederasts'[7] facing trial no longer localised sexuality in the genitals but in the brain. Krafft-Ebing took a strong interest in the legal implications of his psychiatric research findings and believed that science had a role in progressive legal reform. He drew his interest in medical law from his maternal grandfather. Mittermaier had been one of the leading progressive legal minds of his day, and his grandson, though he was pursuing a career in medicine, inherited his grandfather's passion for legal reform.

In 1864, while he was still a medical student, Krafft-Ebing combined his two preoccupations in psychiatry and law, publishing an article on sensory perception and insanity as a medico-legal defence in *Friedreichs Blätter für gerichtlichen Medicin*.[8] It was highly unusual that a newly graduated medical student would gain a foothold in what was then the preeminent journal of forensic medicine, but his grandfather Mittermaier almost certainly pulled strings.[9] The first few paragraphs of his article give a flavour of his early progressive instincts around the role science could play in legal reform:

> Only when the administration of justice stopped appearing like an angel of death with a flaming sword and opened the doors to the results of the

> natural sciences could the endless series of judicial murders, witch trials and persecutions find its end.[10]

Krafft-Ebing's later career showed that he was not just a progressive psychiatrist with an interest in law reform. He was also surprisingly sympathetic to the difficulties encountered by his same-sex attracted patients. Although this therapeutic approach would become a standard among the sexologists in the early twentieth century, it was unusual for a psychiatrist in late nineteenth-century Austria. One reason for Krafft-Ebing's empathetic perspective was a crucially important but now lost correspondence that he maintained with the early queer activist Karl Heinrich Ulrichs. This correspondence spurred Krafft-Ebing's interest in sexual science and mollified his approach to his same-sex attracted patients, but it also directly influenced some of his urning readers to send him unsolicited sexual autobiographies in the decades that followed.

The Ulrichs Connection

Karl Heinrich Ulrichs was a Hanoverian lawyer who wrote twelve pamphlets promulgating a theory of sexuality and arguments for law reform between the years 1864 and 1879. Ulrichs introduced the neologism 'urning' for same sex attracted men and 'dioning' for men attracted to the opposite sex. In 1864, shortly after the publication of his first two pamphlets, Ulrichs discovered Krafft-Ebing's paper in *Friedreichs Blätter*. Ulrichs was delighted with Krafft-Ebing's assertion in favour of progressive legal reform in the article. In his third pamphlet, *Vindicta*, Ulrichs commended Krafft-Ebing's 'splendid essay' and quoted from it approvingly.[11] Shortly after that, it seems that Ulrichs wrote to Krafft-Ebing and probably enclosed one or more of his pamphlets in the letter. They both soon found common ground. While Krafft-Ebing was a doctor with a deep interest in the law, Ulrichs was a lawyer with a deep interest in medicine.[12] The correspondence between the two men would last from 1866 right up to 1894, the year before Ulrichs's death.

Krafft-Ebing was not the only doctor Ulrichs lobbied, though he is the only one with whom he maintained a lifelong epistolary connection. Ulrichs distributed his pamphlets in a deliberate lobbying campaign to the leading medical researchers of his day. Griesinger may even have been one of Ulrichs's medical targets. In 1868, Griesinger made his first comment in print about sexual orientation to the same sex when he redefined it as a constitutional pathology.[13] Griesinger died only a few months later, after contracting diphtheria following an appendix operation. He was succeeded by his deputy, Carl Westphal, who most certainly was a recipient of Ulrichs's lobbying. Westphal had read and absorbed Ulrichs's works when he decided to convene a seminar at the Charité to discuss the subject. On 15 December 1868, the Berlin Medical Psychology Society met to discuss the psychiatry of sexuality including Ulrichs's ideas.[14] Only a couple of months later, Westphal published a research paper with two case studies, one same-sex attracted woman with depression and a male crossdressing sex worker with epilepsy.[15] This is the paper that Foucault later credited as the 'date of birth' of homosexuality.[16] Westphal didn't use Ulrichs's terminology, preferring his own neologism *conträre Sexualempfindung* (contrary sexual feeling), but he quoted him extensively, and his theory owed much to Ulrichs's own outline of the urning. Unlike Ulrichs, but in line with new psychiatry, Westphal located the aetiology of contrary sexual feeling in a pathological process resulting from hereditary degeneration.

In the decade that followed, research psychiatry embedded pathological contrary sexual feeling as a resilient and widely accepted scientific model. Westphal's paper inspired other psychiatrists to approach the subject and publish their own pathologising case studies.[17] Within months, psychiatrists overseas had translated Westphal's neologism *conträre Sexualempfindung* into English as 'contrary sexual feeling/instinct' and papers started appearing in other languages.[18] Ulrichs's intervention had embedded an ontological turn right at the inception of serious psychiatric research. This was a big step forward in the scientific study of sexuality. The urning identity that Ulrichs had originally described in 1864 had become a psychiatric category by the 1870s, a point noted in a letter sent to Ulrichs by a forensic examiner in Hamburg:

> You may rightfully point to the fact that your publications have had a significant effect on shaking the false belief that vice and wickedness always have been at the root in the one in whom these perverse drives appear. Under the term 'contrary sexual feeling', the fact which you emphasise, i.e., the fact of the congenital nature of that drive, has been assumed as absolute by the other side.[19]

Ulrichs's lobbying had captured the attention of psychiatry, which went on to colonise the study of human sexuality in Germany, largely using the framework he had established. However, in the process it had reduced the happy, healthy urning to a contra-sexual beset by a pathological condition caused by hereditary degeneration. Psychiatrists accepted that the law should change, but only if the contra-sexual became a subject for their therapeutic interventions.

Krafft-Ebing published his own first contribution to the burgeoning field of sexual science in 1877 in Westphal's *Archiv für Psychiatrie und Nervenkrankheiten*.[20] This paper surveyed all the psychiatric and forensic research to date, including Ulrichs's works, and presented three new case studies. Krafft-Ebing sent Ulrichs the manuscript of this paper with a letter acknowledging the intellectual debt he owed the activist:

> From that day when you sent your writings—I believe it was in 1866—I have turned my full attention to this phenomenon, which was just as puzzling as it was interesting to me; and it was only the knowledge of your books which motivated me to study this highly important area.[21]

Krafft-Ebing's and Ulrichs's mutual respect did not mean that they were in total agreement. There were real differences between their standpoints and once again the conclusion to Krafft-Ebing's paper retained the pathologising framework of his psychiatric contemporaries:

> Contrary sexual feeling, where it is congenital, can be clinically regarded as the partial appearance of a neuropsychopathic, mostly hereditary condition and has the significance of a functional symptom of degeneration.[22]

Just before Ulrichs gave up on his campaign in Germany to leave for Italy in 1879, he provided his followers with an evaluation of the progress that had been made in the psychiatric evaluation of the urning cause.[23] Ulrichs noted that psychiatry had 'significantly come closer to my viewpoint' and quoted Krafft-Ebing's letter of acknowledgement. Ulrichs's promotion of Krafft-Ebing at this juncture was significant, though he had no illusions about the real differences between their respective positions:

> We of course do not agree absolutely with each other. To me, Uranism is a physiological, i.e., a hermaphroditic phenomenon, a fact of natural law. Krafft-Ebing, on the other hand, declares it to be something pathological, a manifestation of a disease without, of course, denying its inborn nature.[24]

While Ulrichs mentioned other psychiatrists in this passage, the prominence given to Krafft-Ebing may have led some of his followers to start tracking Krafft-Ebing's publications from that point on.

Krafft-Ebing's Published Works Prior to *Psychopathia Sexualis*

When Krafft-Ebing started writing about sexuality, his two most salient influences in that endeavour, Griesinger's psychiatric degeneration theory and Ulrichs's urning emancipation, were apparently at odds. The disparity between his scientific discipline and the sympathy he had for his same-sex attracted patients, so apparent when he started writing, would begin to resolve through his works in the years that followed.

Ulrichs criticised the psychiatric approach in 1879, writing that it tended to be based on observations on 'urnings who were in institutions for the mentally ill'.[25] This was true of Krafft-Ebing as his experience up to that point had been entirely institutional. His first psychiatric position began at the Illenau asylum in Baden and by 1879 he was director of the Feldhof asylum near Graz in Austria.[26] Krafft-Ebing resigned from the Feldhof in 1880 to focus on his academic position at the University of Graz and a small private clinic he had in the same city.[27] He would also go on, in 1886, to open the upmarket Mariagrün sanatorium in suburban Graz.[28] From this point on, the patients he saw were largely free of major psychiatric problems and came from the higher ranks of society, closer to Krafft-Ebing's own class.[29] Krafft-Ebing was now able to study his patients' sexual conditions without occlusion by accompanying psychopathological conditions.

In 1882, he published the first case studies of same-sex attracted men from this new patient group: two aristocrats and a writer/private tutor with a Doctor of Philosophy.[30] Although one of these patients was seeking therapeutic interventions to modify his sexuality, two of them pointedly were not. The first, Count Z., a thirty-seven-year-old aristocrat, had been troubled by neurasthenia[31] and may have been referred to Krafft-Ebing by relatives. Krafft-Ebing was particularly impressed by the character and appearance of this patient and, when he indicated that he was sexually attracted to his own sex, Krafft-Ebing was sympathetic:

> The patient is neither unhappy about the reversal of his sexual sensation, nor is he able to recognise it as a pathological one. He is all the less able to do so because he feels morally uplifted, happy and relieved by contact with men. How could that be morbid which makes a man happy and inspires him to beauty and nobility! His only misfortune was that social barriers and penal regulations stood in the way of the 'natural' expression of his impulse. This is a great hardship.[32]

Although Count Z. made his case with consummate delicacy, he was nevertheless rejecting Krafft-Ebing's assessment that contrary sexual sensation was a neuropsychological, mostly hereditary, pathological condition. The second case study made the same claim with far less delicacy. G. Dr phil. was a fifty-year-old writer/tutor who had been referred to Krafft-Ebing by the police after being caught in flagrante with a soldier. G. had been living in Italy and was apparently highly educated, though Krafft-Ebing seemed to take a dislike to him, calling him a 'vagabond', 'crazy' and 'madman'. Apparently, G. was well-versed in Ulrichs's theories and acknowledged his urning nature 'which he regards as abnormal but can by no means recognize as pathological'.[33] G. also paraphrased Pausanias's speech from Plato's Symposium, the passage that Ulrichs had used as the source of his 'urning' terminology:

> He thinks that there is nothing left for him and his comrades but to elevate the unnatural that dwells in them to the supernatural. He recognises urning love as the higher, ideal, as the god-like, abstracted love. ... For the justification and explanation of his abnormal sexual sensation, G. draws on Plato 'who was certainly no filthy swine'. Plato already made the allegorical statement that people used to be spheres; the gods separated them into two slices. Mostly man fits on woman, but sometimes also man on man.[34]

Since all the case studies were written by Krafft-Ebing, it is curious that he made a particular effort to record the dissent of Count Z. and G. These men both denied any pathological interpretation of their sexual inclinations. In the discussion that followed, Krafft-Ebing made no direct reference to the fact these two individuals had challenged his theory and instead asserted that 'contrary sexual sensation is not a physiological but a pathological phenomenon'.[35] This juxtaposition of orthodox degeneration theory with unchallenged dissenting case studies lends this paper an ambivalent character—something that would become a feature of all his publications on the subject from that point on.

In Krafft-Ebing's next paper, he tried something different. One of his clinic patients, a Hungarian businessman he called 'Mr X.', had originally consulted Krafft-Ebing about neurasthenia and insomnia. During the clinical interview, Mr X. revealed that he was same-sex attracted, so Krafft-Ebing suggested he write his own account of his sexuality. This autobiographical account is the first of the case studies presented in this book (2.1).[36] Krafft-Ebing published this case study in 1883 in the second edition of a psychiatric textbook.[37] This first autobiography established a trend for unsolicited letter autobiographies in its wake and can be regarded as the prototype sexual autobiography in this series. For urnings following Krafft-Ebing's works, they had first witnessed Krafft-Ebing's tolerance of a dissenting discourse that denied pathologising conclusions and then his deployment of autobiography in a case study. This inspired some of his urning readers to start sending Krafft-Ebing their own sexual life stories.

1.2 The Case Studies

Krafft-Ebing began publishing unsolicited letter autobiographies in three papers published between 1883 and 1885 (2.1, 3.1–3.3).[38] In 1886, he published his first edition of his most important work, *Psychopathia Sexualis*, a book that was expanded and republished by him in eleven editions with the last edition edited by him in 1901.[39] Krafft-Ebing also published supplements entitled *Neue Forschungen auf dem Gebiet der Psychopathia Sexualis* in 1890, 1891 and 1901.[40] One extremely long autobiographical letter combined with a polemic appeared as a paper in *Friedreichs Blätter für gerichtliche Medicin* in 1891 and was republished in modified form in the *Wiener medizinische Blätter* in 1892.[41] These were the publications in which the sexual autobiographies appeared.

Table 1.1 shows the clinical and autobiographical case studies for same-sex attracted men and women within each of the editions of *Psychopathia Sexualis* plus the additional publications from 1882 onwards. In total, there were 410 individual 'contra-sexual' case studies in these publications: 80% were male and 20% female. Three-quarters were clinical accounts of patients visiting his clinical practice or the sanatorium. Krafft-Ebing included self-penned autobiographical case studies, comprising a quarter of all the case studies presented, in every edition of *Psychopathia Sexualis* from 1886 to 1901. However, he reused some case studies in several different editions and borrowed case studies from the publications of other psychiatrists. Filtering out repeats and borrowings, there were 130 original case studies of which 107 were of men and 23 of women. Of these, 89 were case studies written by the clinician in his practice (71 men and 18 women), while 34 were autobiographical case studies of men and five were clinical case studies of women that included autobiographical content. A further two were polemic letters sent in by urning men. Although there were no unsolicited letter autobiographies from women, Krafft-Ebing encouraged five of his women patients, including the passing man Sandor V, to write about their sexual selves. Krafft-Ebing then

Table 1.1 The case studies in Richard von Krafft-Ebing's works from 1882 up to his death in 1902[42]

				Novel case studies		
	Total	*Gender split*	*Autobiogs*	*Total novel case studies*	*Clinical*	*Autobiogs*
AZfP. 1882[a]	3	3M	0	3M	3M	0
Lehrb. 1883[b]	4	4M	1M	4M	3M	1M
Irrenf. 1884[c]	6	5M, 1F	1M	5M, 1F	4M, 1F	1M
JfP. 1885[d]	2	2M	2M	2M	0	2M
			Psychopathia Sexualis			
PS 1886 (1st ed.)	3	2M, 1F	1M	1M, 1F	1F	1M
PS 1887 (2nd ed.)	14	12M, 2F	5M	8M, 1F	5M, 1F	3M
PS 1888 (3rd ed.)	22	19M, 3F	10M	8M	3M	5M
PS 1889 (4th ed.)	43	35M, 8F	13M, 2F	11M, 4F	8M, 2F	3M, 2F[i]
PS 1890 (5th ed.)	60	53M, 7F	18 M, 3F	17M, 1F	12M	5M, 1F
1890X[e]	13	12M, 1F	6M	12M, 1F	6M 1F	6M
PS 1891 (6th ed.)	34	28M, 6F	15M, 2F	1M	0	1M
1891X[f]	12	11M, 2F	6M	4M, 1F	1F	4M
1891/1892[g]	1	1M	1M	1M	0	1M[j]
PS 1892 (7th ed.)	52	41M, 11F	16M	6M, 2F	3M, 2F	3M
PS 1893 (8th ed.)	50	39M, 11F	16M, 3F	0	0	0
PS 1894 (9th ed.)	40	25M, 15F	10M, 4F	5F	4F	1F
PS 1898 (10th ed.)	38	25M, 13F	6M, 5F	6M, 1F	6M	1F
PS 1901 (11th ed.)	36	23M 13F	1M, 3F	13M, 1F	13M	0
1901X[h]	11	7M 4F	0	5M, 4F	5M, 4F	0
TOTALS	410	318M 92F	113M, 22F	107M, 18F	71M, 23F	36M, 5F

(*continued*)

Table 1.1 (continued)

[a]Richard von Krafft-Ebing, 'Zur "conträren Sexualempfindung" in klinisch-forensischer Hinsicht', *Allgemeine Zeitschrift für Psychiatrie* 38 (1882): 211–27

[b]Richard von Krafft-Ebing, *Lehrbuch der Psychiatrie auf klinischer Grundlage für practische Ärzte und Studirende*, 2nd ed. (Stuttgart: Ferdinand Enke, 1883)

[c]Richard von Krafft-Ebing, 'Zur Lehre von der conträren Sexualempfindung', *Der Irrenfreund* 26 (1884): 1–14

[d]Richard von Krafft-Ebing, 'Die conträre Sexualempfindung vor dem Forum', *Jarbücher für Psychiatrie* 6 (1885): 34–47

[e]Richard von Krafft-Ebing, *Neue Forschungen auf dem Gebiet der Psychopathia Sexualis: Eine medicinisch-psychologische Studie* (Stuttgart: Ferdinand Enke, 1890)

[f]Richard von Krafft-Ebing, *Neue Forschungen auf dem Gebiet der Psychopathia Sexualis: Eine medicinisch-psychologische Studie* (Stuttgart: Ferdinand Enke, 1891)

[g]Richard von Krafft-Ebing, 'Zur conträren Sexualempfindung: Autobiographie und strafrechtliche Betrachtungen über den Paragraphen 175 des deutschen Strafgesetzbuchs von einem Conträr-Sexualen', *Friedreichs Blätter für gerichtliche Medicin* 42 (1891): 385–400; Richard von Krafft-Ebing, 'Zur conträren Sexualempfindung: Autobiographie und strafrechtliche Betrachtungen von einem conträr Sexualen', *Wiener medizinische Blätter* 15 (1892): 42–4

[h]Richard von Krafft-Ebing, 'Neue Forschungen auf dem Gebiet der Psychopathia Sexualis', *Jahrbuch für sexuelle Zwischenstufen* 3 (1901): 1–36

[i]Includes polemic letter from John Addington Symonds

[j]Combined sexual case history and legal polemic

included sections from these accounts in the case studies he subsequently published. These 41 case studies are the subject of the foregoing discussion and are published in translation in this volume.

For the purposes of this book, the autobiographic case studies have been sorted into nine categories. These are not the categories that Krafft-Ebing used. From 1889 on, Krafft-Ebing grouped his contra-sexual case studies under four broad headings.[43] He did not separate the sexes but classified his case studies into individuals who were attracted to both sexes, those who were solely same-sex attracted, and effeminate men/masculine women or individuals who physically resembled the opposite sex. Krafft-Ebing's categories were porous and imprecise and related to the therapeutic approaches used in his clinic. Most of the nine categories used in this book focus instead on the purpose of the author in writing the sexual autobiography. The first case study (*The First Autobiography*) is in a category of its own, as it was commissioned by Krafft-Ebing from a man undergoing treatment in his clinic in the early 1880s. The next three case-study categories (*Dissenters*; *Two Polemics*; *For the Good of Science*) were unsolicited letter autobiographies, with all of them coming from same-sex attracted men with no stated intention of seeking a cure. The *Dissenters* category comprises ten individuals who disputed pathologisation; the *Two*

Polemics are two long letters expounding political and legal arguments for sexual law reform; and *For the Good of Science* presents seven men who wrote to Krafft-Ebing with their sexual life stories in the hope that it would contribute to a better scientific understanding of their condition.

The next two categories (*The Women; Gender Nonconformity*) relate to individuals whose personal characteristics and purpose in writing was distinct from all the other groups. *The Women* comprises four partial case studies from women, and *Gender Nonconformity* details three case studies of individuals whose degree of gender nonconformity anticipates more modern categories of trans men and women.

The final three sections (*Pathologisers; Psychic Hermaphrodites; In Search of a Cure*) all relate to men more disposed to therapeutic intervention. *Pathologisers* includes seven same-sex attracted men who accepted their sexuality was a pathological condition; *Psychic Hermaphrodites*, the only Krafft-Ebing category reused in the current subdivision, refers to the men sexually attracted to both sexes who were believed to be the most amenable to therapeutic interventions; and the final category, *In Search of a Cure*, includes two men sexually attracted to both sexes who underwent therapeutic interventions.

The case studies in this book follow the discursive patterns established in nineteenth-century psychiatry in providing descriptions of body features including genital size and shape, mental and physical health, family histories of health and disease, and accounts of life events from childhood to the present. Women's sexual availability to men through prostitution meant that it was not unusual for young Austrian men and some German men to visit the brothel at least once when they came of age.[44] For same-sex attracted men this was a first 'test' of the limits of their sexual desire. A large proportion of the case studies of men in this book, twenty-three out of thirty-six, mentioned a visit to a brothel as they entered manhood. For some, this resulted in an immediate feeling of disgust at the female form. While this reaction can be explained in part by the circumstance of a forced sexual encounter against their natures, some of the accounts veer into prejudice. The misogynistic attitudes towards women among some of the correspondents probably reflected prevailing patriarchal cultural disdain for women in general in late nineteenth-century Europe.

The primary focus of all the autobiographical case studies was an account of the sexual experience of the individual. At least for same-sex attracted men, the articulation of these sexual and relationship histories was not necessarily an unusual thing to do, as one autobiographer noted:

> As soon as contra-sexualists come to know each other, a detailed exchange of their previous experiences, loves and conquests takes place, as far as such a conversation is not excluded by the social differences of both. Only in very few cases this conversation with new acquaintances is omitted. (3.7)[45]

In much the same way that contemporary gay men and women might recount 'coming out stories', these autobiographical tales functioned as a discursive practice that reinforced their authors' sexual identification. In telling their sexual histories, they shared details of their erotic fantasies, masturbatory habits and sexual preferences. In some cases, the writing is so erotically charged that when reproducing the case studies for publication, Krafft-Ebing rendered the more explicit descriptions in Latin.

The Dissenters and Their Followers

Possibly the most eye-catching case studies in Krafft-Ebing's works are the ones that openly challenged his pathologising conclusions. There were ten of these case studies plus a further two polemic letters that also challenged Krafft-Ebing's conclusions. Krafft-Ebing was under no obligation to publish these accounts and it was certainly within his power to edit out any dissenting statements if he had so desired.[46] That he did not do so and instead used these dissenting case studies in repeated volumes suggests he had some sympathy with the sentiment even if he could not voice his own support. Krafft-Ebing's toleration of the dissenting voice and his frequent appeals for letter autobiographies generated a steady flow of sexual autobiographies from other followers of his works. In so doing, the pages of *Psychopathia Sexualis* became, for these men, a platform for negotiating the parameters of sexual orientation.

Krafft-Ebing published the first three dissenting case studies in 1884 and 1885. It is worth examining these first three because they each reveal the most obvious rejections of pathological explanations. The first of these came from a thirty-eight-year-old masculine German businessman who was one of six case studies that appeared in the journal *Irrenfreund* (3.1).[47] He revealed early on that he was familiar with Ulrichs's pamphlets and had been one of the urnings following Krafft-Ebing's published works. Specifically, he wrote that he had read Krafft-Ebing's 1882 paper in the *Allgemeine Zeitschrift für Psychiatrie* and that he had been impressed by the sympathy Krafft-Ebing showed to dissenting urnings there. This was the first published example of an urning follower of Ulrichs turning to the works of Krafft-Ebing and then contributing with an autobiographical letter for use as a case study. The man had no intention of seeking a cure and, apart from his legal situation and enforced exile, he was quite content with his sexual orientation.

In 1885, Krafft-Ebing reproduced two more autobiographical accounts he had received in unsolicited letters from individuals who rejected any notion of pathology and located their sexual awakening with the works of Ulrichs (3.2, 3.3).[48] The accounts follow the structure and content of Krafft-Ebing's published case studies, which suggests that both urnings had been keen readers of these works. Their letters supplied all the kind of content Krafft-Ebing could easily use. This was not a case of inventing content to fit Krafft-Ebing's theories; if anything, the two urnings intended to persuade Krafft-Ebing he was wrong to pathologise them. However, they had been attentive to the way Krafft-Ebing constructed his case studies and so included details about parental physical and mental illness, masturbation as a teenager or young adult and other features that Krafft-Ebing included in standard clinical evaluations. The first of these case studies came from a well-educated, senior civil servant. Commenting on his mental health, he wrote, 'I cannot find the love for men pathological. I would therefore be psychologically completely healthy were it not for a strange mania that haunts and torments me in my sexual life' (3.2).[49] The mania to which he referred was the relentless drive for sexual satisfaction that he often had to relieve with masturbation. He closed his letter with an appeal:

> When will we be able to approach the matter without prejudice, even in the public arena? In any case, science must not pause for a moment to disseminate the results obtained as far as possible and make them understandable even to the layman.[50]

The second letter case study, from a forty-eight-year-old married urning showed the same concern to proffer his case study to advance scientific research (3.3). This letter contains a strong endorsement of the Ulrichian anti-pathological position:

> It was only when I was about 30 years old that I came across the writings of Numa (Ulrichs) and I cannot describe what a relief it was for me to learn that there were many other men who were just as sexually inclined as I was, and that what I felt sexually was not an aberration but a special sexual disposition inherent in me by nature. For the first time I experienced the pleasure

> of finding sexual satisfaction through direct contact with a man's body. I no longer tried in vain to fight against a deeply implanted disposition. (3.3)[51]

This man did not just attest to his mental health, but also located the origins of his wellbeing with his sexual awakening: '[S]ince I let my urning nature run free, I am happier, healthier and more efficient!' (3.3).[52] The case study gives a strong expression of the liberating experience of finding a name, and with it, a sense of belonging afforded by the urning identity. While they complied with all of Krafft-Ebing's requirements for case-study content, they were also challenging Krafft-Ebing's assumptions and pushing him to change his position. The first three dissenting autobiographers all state clearly their association with Ulrichs and his ideas and their rigid opposition to pathologising conclusions. These men saw themselves as secure and happy in their urning natures and rejected any suggestion that disease or hereditary taint played a part. Nor did they see any point in changing their sexual dispositions. In his preamble to the 1885 study, Krafft-Ebing speculated that some urnings, possibly a minority, could be mentally healthy.[53] He also appealed for more letter autobiographies. This prompted seven more urning readers to do the same as these first three. In total, there were ten dissenting case studies and two accounts that eschewed autobiography to make direct polemic arguments for reform.

Table 1.2 displays the year the case study appeared and the number of times it was repeated, the occupation of the author, his age and the terminology he used about himself. Most of the men either directly mentioned a connection with Ulrichs or his writings or showed familiarity with his principal arguments. They were mostly old enough to remember the period when Ulrichs's campaign was active. The one exception is the medical student in his twenties (3.5).[54] He wrote that he had been inspired by reading the case studies in *Psychopathia Sexualis*, rather than Ulrichs's pamphlets.

The ten dissenting case studies make a trenchant case for revision of the psychiatric category. It is remarkable that Krafft-Ebing was apparently happy to publish these dissenting case studies alongside clinical case studies of men seeking therapeutic intervention. Most of the case studies were printed more than once, but there was one dissenting case study, in particular, that was repeated five further times. This one was a highly sexed medical man who was so outspoken on his sexual exploits that Krafft-Ebing had to render substantial parts of these descriptions in Latin (3.7).[55] This case study first appeared in the 1890 edition and then all but one subsequent edition.

Table 1.2 Characteristics of the men who wrote dissenting autobiographies and the two who wrote polemics

Case study number	*Year published (repeated?)*	*Occupation*	*Age*	*Terminology*
3.1	1884 (2)	Unstated	40s?	Urning
3.2	1885 (2)	Civil servant	35	Urning
3.3	1885 (2)	Independently wealthy, scientific writer	48	Urning
3.4	1888 (3)	Soldier, businessman	50	Urning, contra-sexual
3.5	1890 (1)	Medical student	20s?	Urning
3.6	1890 (3)	Merchant and owner of small shop	Early 30s	Urning
3.7	1890 (5)	Medical doctor		Contra-sexual
3.8	1890 (0)	World traveller	36	Contra-sexual, urning
3.9	1890 (0)	Concert musician	34	Contra-sexual
3.10	1891 (2)	Engineer	37	Contra-sexual, urning.
4.1	1890 (1)	[John Addington Symonds—English writer]	50	Urning
4.2	1891 (1)	Senior civil servant	45	Contrary sexual, homosexual and urning

The final two items in Table 1.2 are two letters that largely dispensed with biographic details to mount polemic defences of the urning lifestyle and arguments for legislative reform. The first of these (4.1)[56] came from John Addington Symonds, a prominent English writer and latterly a proponent of homosexual emancipation, then resident in Davos, Switzerland.[57] The interesting thing about Symonds's letter is that despite presenting as an urning, struggling to exist in a hostile world, Symonds had no direct experience of living as or calling himself an urning. When he wrote the letter in mid-1889, he had only just encountered the writings of Ulrichs and Krafft-Ebing so the letter is a 'thought exercise' inspired by what he had read of the lives of urnings. The second polemic is a long legal disquisition on the rights and wrongs of criminalising same-sex sexuality written by a senior civil servant (4.2).[58] Krafft-Ebing was particularly impressed by this man's arguments, though the legalistic nature of the writing can be a little impenetrable to those unfamiliar with German jurisprudence.

At least for those who could access them, the presence of autobiographical case studies in Krafft-Ebing's works also served an educative

Table 1.3 Characteristics of the men who wrote to Krafft-Ebing 'for the good of science'

Case study number	*Year published (repeated?)*	*Occupation*	*Age*	*Terminology*
5.1	1886 (8)	Military doctor	40	Urning
5.2	1887 (4)	Factory official		Urning
5.3	1887 (1)			Contra-sexual, homosexual
5.4	1887 (2)	Medical doctor/ military doctor		None
5.5	1888 (7)	Merchant	34.5	Urning
5.6	1889 (1)	Lawyer	27	None
5.7	1890 (1)	Civil servant with small income	39	None

purpose. Table 1.3 includes seven case studies from men who wrote to Krafft-Ebing 'for the good of science'.

These case studies were less purposely deviating from Krafft-Ebing's thesis, though none of them voiced any acceptance of pathologising conclusions. As such, they can be considered to be part of the urning platform of autobiographic negotiation that was playing out in successive editions of *Psychopathia Sexualis.*

Three of these uncomplicated case studies supplied 'for the good of science' were presumably so well thought of that Krafft-Ebing used them multiple times. The most republished autobiography of all was a letter from another sexually ambitious married forty-year-old medical doctor who was a masculine urning (5.1).[59] Krafft-Ebing used this case study in the first edition of *Psychopathia Sexualis* and then repeated it in every single one of the next eight editions up to 1894. Similarly, the case study of an effeminate thirty-four-year-old merchant was deployed in every single edition between 1888 and 1898 (5.5).[60] Another multiply repeated urning autobiography came from a factory official who had experienced many unrequited loves but recounts his introduction one night to the urning social scene where he experienced 'cheerfulness, exuberance and carefree enjoyment of life' (5.2).[61]

While a majority of the men who wrote dissenting letters, polemics or wrote 'for the good of science' used the word urning to describe themselves (10 out of 19), they were also more likely to use other terms. Seven case studies used the psychiatric term 'contra-sexual' either in conjunction with the urning terminology or alone. It was one of these case studies that, in 1887, also introduced the word 'homosexual' for the first time (5.3)[62] Although Krafft-Ebing started using the homosexual terminology himself from 1889 onwards, there is only one of the letters in this group, from the second polemicist, that used the word 'homosexual' (4.2). Even there, the author did so while using the words 'urning and 'contra-sexual' as well.

The men who wrote to Krafft-Ebing to prove their good health or for the good of science were surprisingly open about their sexual practices but displayed the common prejudices against certain sexual acts that reflected widely held social attitudes of the time. Partly because of the legal prohibition, they mostly did not practice pederasty (anal intercourse) widely. There were only four out of nineteen autobiographies that mentioned active or passive anal intercourse (2.4, 2.8, 5.1 and 5.4) and many of the other autobiographers regarded it as disgusting, taking great care to distance their own sexual practice from it. For instance, one correspondent argued for

> some way by which the great multitude can be taught a milder and more reasonable judgment of it [contra-sexual feeling], above all the one thing at least, that one does not regard contra-sexual feeling as synonymous with pederasty, as is unfortunately done by most, I should like to say by all. (3.10)[63]

It is possible that pederasty was more prevalent but underreported due to shame and stigma. Instead, the sexually active autobiographers described practicing mutual masturbation and, to a lesser degree, oral or interfemoral sex.

Many of the correspondents believed, along with psychiatrists, that masturbation weakened the individual and caused mental and physical illness. Abstention entirely from masturbation, though recommended at the time, was an option only one or two followed. For example, a thirty-nine-year-old married Hungarian civil servant, who described his sexual awakening with other men as an 'enlightenment', wrote of masturbation: 'I did not masturbate either in the unenlightened or later in the enlightened state, and that my relative well-being can perhaps be traced back to this state' (5.7).[64] The entrenched disapproval of masturbation in medicine led some correspondents to argue that it was healthier to engage in mutual masturbation and other sexual practices than it was to masturbate alone. Mutual masturbation was the most prevalent sexual practice among the male autobiographers. In Germany this was one sexual practice between men that was not regarded as criminal. Krafft-Ebing later wrote that he regarded mutual masturbation as healthy and preferable to pathogenic solitary masturbation.[65]

The age stratification of sexual objects is also something worth noting. Homosexual acts were illegal in both Austria and Germany and the age of heterosexual consent in both nations was 14. Most of the urning men who stated their ideal partner type where an age was stated were attracted to men their own age or slightly younger. Some older urnings had a hankering after young men but in most cases the stated ages were mindful of the age of consent as a legal boundary. However, there were one or two whose interests were in teenage boys below the age of consent around puberty. One man stated he was attracted to 'boys of at least 10, but mostly towards young boys of 15–20' (3.6).[66] He had not consummated these desires but satisfied the urge by secretly masturbating in close proximity to teenagers he was attracted to. Another individual who was sexually active indicated that he was interested only in boys 12–16 (3.5).[67] Hellenistic age-stratified same-sex relations would later be championed by the masculists in Berlin but among the autobiographers these practices do not appear to have been widespread.

These autobiographical urning case studies supplied in dissent or for the good of science form a corpus of urning outreach. They made up the majority of the male autobiographies (19 out of 36) and, since they were more likely to be repeated, they constituted an eye-catching component of every single edition of *Psychopathia Sexualis*. As such, these case studies are evidence of a remarkable joint endeavour to appropriately codify and qualify the urning in the psychiatric literature. This meant that the urnings who participated in this, and the wider audience of urnings reading *Psychopathia Sexualis*, were inclined to see Krafft-Ebing as an ally in the urning cause.

The Women

Relatively speaking, female sexuality was a mostly undeveloped component of Krafft-Ebing's evolving sexology.[68] Sexually inverted women had been the subjects of psychiatric enquiry since Westphal's seminal paper in 1869, but there is no evidence in the nineteenth century of women in the German-speaking world volunteering sexual autobiographies.[69] There has been no recorded evidence of any intersection of advocacy similar to that seen between urnings and Krafft-Ebing for same-sex attracted women and psychiatry in this period.

Of the twenty-three women described in clinical case studies in *Psychopathia Sexualis*, all were visitors to Krafft-Ebing's clinic or resided in his sanatorium. Since lesbianism was illegal in Austria, they either sought cures from Krafft-Ebing or were committed to his therapeutic regime by relatives or the authorities. In four cases, Krafft-Ebing encouraged his female patients to supply sexual autobiographies. Unlike the cases where Krafft-Ebing used autobiographies from his male patients, Krafft-Ebing only published part of each woman's autobiography and preferred to paraphrase the rest. This was perhaps a trope of an era when all doctors were male and the understanding of or appreciation of female psychology was lacking. Whether or not Krafft-Ebing embodied this prejudice, there was clearly not the same level of mutual trust when it came to his female patients. In 1898, he wrote about his same-sex-attracted female patients:

> Concerning the occurrence of homosexual feelings in women, the present science has much more scanty observations at its disposal than concerning this anomaly in men. It would be unjustified to draw from this the conclusion that contra-sexual sensation is rarer in women, because if it is really a functional degenerative phenomenon, degenerative influences will be just as strong in women as in men.[70]

Krafft-Ebing used the words contra-sexual and homosexual to describe his female patients, but Table 1.4 shows that none of the women who supplied autobiographies used any word to describe their sexual dispositions.

All four of these women had been referred to Krafft-Ebing by relatives or the authorities. Both of the women in service, as a maid (6.2)[71] and as

Table 1.4 Characteristics of the women who supplied autobiographies at Krafft-Ebing's request

Case study number	*Year published (repeated?)*	*Occupation*	*Age*	*Terminology*
6.1	1889 (5)	Ilma S., daughter of a merchant	29	None
6.2	1889 (7)	C. R., maid	26	None
6.3	1894 (2)	Miss L., governess	55	None
6.4	1898 (1)	Miss X.	22	None

a governess (6.3),[72] seem to have been referred to Krafft-Ebing as a consequence of criminal proceedings following the seduction of female members of the families they were working for. Two of the women reported periodic transvestism, partly as an expression of their masculine personalities but also for employment purposes (6.1, 6.2).[73] The effects of widespread male cultural disdain for women were also revealed in these case studies. Two of the women attributed their sexual alienation to having traumatically witnessed men sexually assaulting other women in what Krafft-Ebing described as 'acquired' contra-sexuality. C. R., a 26-year-old housemaid passing as a man for employment purposes, was expected to visit brothels with her male colleagues as a matter of course and listen to their course language (6.1).[74] These experiences of heterosexual male culture, compounded with her witnessing the poor behaviour of her male cousin, were all so disgusting to her that she stopped passing as a man. Miss X. claimed that witnessing sexual violence was a causative factor in her evolving sexuality (6.4).[75] Only two of these accounts mention sexual acts: mutual masturbation (6.3)[76] and cunnilingus (6.4).[77] If anything, the autobiographies from these women seem more sensuous than sensual and it was relationships, rather than casual sex, that ordered their accounts. Whether that underlined a critical difference between female and male sexual selfhood in the late nineteenth century cannot be ascertained with such a small sample. Perhaps because there were so few of them, the four fragmented case studies from women were more likely to be repeated in subsequent editions. Two of these were highly republished: the case study of Ilma S., a 29-year-old daughter of a wealthy merchant, appeared for the first time in 1889 and was repeated in five subsequent volumes (6.1)[78]; the housemaid 'C. R.', referred to above, was first published in 1889 and then repeated in every single edition after that (6.2).[79]

The women that Krafft-Ebing extracted autobiographies from were perhaps atypical as they did not display the same strongly asserted sexual-self seen in the male autobiographies. However, there were other case studies of women, without autobiographic elements, where the women were unmarried, independent and appeared to be expressing a fully developed sexual identity. Some wore their hair short and wore masculine cuts to their clothing. Krafft-Ebing described a thirty-eight-year-old Austrian woman, referred by relatives who suspected she had sexual interest in women after she refused an offer of marriage:

> Already at the first meeting the patient made a striking impression by her dress, features and demeanour. She wore a man's hat, her hair cropped short, pince-nez, masculine cravats, a jacket-like upper dress with a masculine cut reaching far down over the lady's dress, boots with heels.[80]

Even the younger patients could have a keen sense of what they believed were their sexual rights. A Viennese family had committed an eighteen-year-old called Elsa to Krafft-Ebing's sanatorium because the forced separation from her nineteen-year-old friend Fransziska had left her in profound distress. Krafft-Ebing was surprised the next day when

> Fransziska came storming into my private apartment in order to obtain my consent to reunite with her beloved, possibly to force the liberation of her friend from her captivity with the help of the courts![81]

These are just fragments, but they give a flavour of what was possibly an early published window into lesbian lifestyles in the German-speaking world in the 1880s and 1890s.

Gender Nonconformists

Whereas many of his predecessors conflated gender identity and sexual object choice under a single category, Krafft-Ebing now presented the urning/homosexual as a distinct subtype from hyper-effeminacy in men, hyper-masculinity in women and androgyny/gynandry.[82] However, he still saw them as directly related to each other. There were three case studies of gender nonconforming subjects that were either letter autobiographies or included autobiographical elements. Probably the most famous of these was the case study of Count Sandor (Charlotte Sarolta Vay), a 'passing man' from Hungary who had married a Viennese heiress but was subsequently discovered not to be who he said he was (7.1).[83] The society scandal resulted in a criminal court case where Krafft-Ebing spoke in defence and Sandor gave a rousing speech that concluded: 'God has given me love in my heart. If he created me like this and not otherwise, am I to blame for it, or are the eternally unfathomable ways of fate?'[84] Sandor was acquitted and returned to Hungary. The other two case studies in this section are two full-letter autobiographies from men reporting two kinds of acute and chronic gender dysphoria. The first, a medical student of twenty-two, wrote in 1890 of his fervent desire to live his life as a woman (7.2).[85]

Table 1.5 Characteristics of three gender nonconforming autobiographers

Case study number	*Year published (repeated?)*	*Occupation*	*Age*	*Terminology*
7.1	1890 (5)	Sarolta (Charlotte) Countess V./ Count Sandor, aristocrat and writer	30	None
7.2	1890 (3)	Medical student	22	None
7.3	1890 (4)	Obstetrician	48	None

The second, a long account by a forty-eight-year-old married obstetrician, detailed a progressive and almost psychotic dysphoria where they had the sensation that their body had become entirely female (7.3).[86]

Table 1.5 presents the characteristics of these three case studies. Like the women, these individuals did not use any of the available terms to describe themselves. While Sarolta and the medical student were ostensibly same-sex attracted, the obstetrician had a wife and reported no same-sex desire. However, in both the student and the obstetrician, sexual desire was muted and not self-regarded as an organising principle. It was gender identification that predominated as the definitive characteristic in all three of these cases. Notably, after Sandor's acquittal, he continued to live as a man. At this point in time, psychiatry had very little to offer these individuals other than to record their characteristics and predicaments. It would be another two decades before Magnus Hirschfeld and colleagues started negotiating practical solutions for transvestite Germans.[87] The full resolution of this conflation of sexuality and cross-gender identification did not come until the early twentieth century when Havelock Ellis described 'Eonism' as a separate category and Magnus Hirschfeld rebadged it as 'transsexual'.[88]

Perhaps because these three autobiographies came from underreported groups, they were more likely to be repeatedly published. This was particularly true of Count Sandor's case, first deployed in 1890 and then repeated five more times. The rather lurid account of the obstetrician also appeared for the first time in 1890 and was repeated four more times.

Pathologisers

Those who accepted the pathologising arguments were not a homogeneous group. Three of them admitted their sexualities were pathological but were not seeking any therapeutic intervention (8.1, 8.4 and 8.7).[89]

This curious self-conception may have been a strategic position taken by some urning advocates. In 1891, the sexologist Albert Moll overheard and reported a discussion between N. N. (the author and activist Adolf Glaser) and a friend:

> N. N., a thoroughly objective, calm gentleman, said to X: 'If only we could at least get it accepted that the contrary sexual sensation is considered pathological, so that we are no longer considered criminals.' X replied: 'I can never agree to that; I would rather choose the present state. We are quite simply outvoted by the rest, and if they do consider the affection to be a disease, then it would land us all in the madhouse.'[90]

At the time, Krafft-Ebing was advocating repeal of the anti-sodomy laws in Austria and Germany, a position he shared with several of his psychiatric peers. Some urnings may have been so directly influenced by reading these calls that they aligned their self-conceptions with the pathologising theories of their psychiatric ally, Krafft-Ebing.

The other four autobiographies came from urnings who were highly distressed about their conditions, regarded themselves as diseased and sought therapeutic intervention. Their desire to change was unlikely to be satisfied as Krafft-Ebing did not accept that congenital urnings, those born that way and solely attracted to their own sex, were amenable to therapeutic intervention. In the first 1886 edition of *Psychopathia Sexualis*, he had written:

> The possibility asserted by Tarnowsky (op. cit. p. 17 u. flP.) that a real urning with a congenital perversion of the sexual life can be freed from his pathological sexual direction by education and brought to normal sexual sensation, I must deny on the basis of my experience.[91]

In these cases, therapeutic interventions could only focus on educating the patient towards abstinence, alleviating psychiatric comorbidities or curing addictions to masturbation.

Table 1.6 shows that all but one of these men used the word 'urning' about themselves. Two of them reported suicidal ideation (8.3, 8.5)[92] and two were so distressed by their sexual nature that they tried to suppress it (8.2, 8.4).[93] Two of them had read about the therapeutic interventions Krafft-Ebing had used with other patients and asked for the same, with one citing his experience with Carl Hansen, the stage hypnotist (8.5, 8.6).[94] Krafft-Ebing did not indicate whether any of these men visited his clinic.

Table 1.6 Characteristics of urnings who accepted pathologisation

Case study number	*Year published (repeated?)*	*Occupation*	*Age*	*Terminology*
8.1	1888 (0)	Landowner with a country estate	Around 40	Urning
8.2	1888 (3)	Educator	Late 40s (46?)	Contra-sexual, urning
8.3	1888 (0)		27	Urning
8.4	1889 (1)	Actor	20s	Urning
8.5	1890 (1)		33	Urning
8.6	1891 (2)	Estate manager (forester)	33 (but later talks of being 38)	Contra-sexual, urning
8.7	1891 (2)	Responsible profession	38	None

Sexually, these men were less likely to be at ease with their sexualities. Some men feared the consequences and, so afraid of the law, abstained from both masturbation and sex. This could lead to embarrassing consequences, as one desperate middle-aged man recounted:

> When the doctor examined my genitals, erection occurred immediately, it seized me like a dizziness, I fell around the doctor's neck and there was an outpouring of semen. The doctor laughed and said that I needed nothing more than a woman. (8.2)[95]

Even if they did not see masturbation as the cause of their perverse feelings, some still saw it as magnifying the problem: 'I believe that masturbation has inflamed the innate feeling to blazing embers' (8.7).[96] These correspondents revealed deep feelings of disgust and self-loathing when discussing masturbation and their struggle, in vain, against it. Notably, this group of case studies was less likely to be republished than any other group of case studies.

Psychic Hermaphrodites

Krafft-Ebing classified individuals attracted to both sexes as '*Psychische Hermaphrodisie*' (Psychic or Mental Hermaphrodisia) and initially made a distinction between those he considered to be congenitally directed to both sexes and those that had an acquired sexual disposition:

> In the case of (congenital) psychic hermaphrodisia, the *vita sexualis* always debuts in the homosexual direction, which is far more strongly predisposed; in the case of acquired contrary sexual feeling, the debut is in the heterosexual and the homosexual inclination appears and develops on the basis of tangible occasional causes (masturbatory neurasthenia, psychic moments).[97]

Krafft-Ebing believed that the men and women with an acquired disposition towards both sexes were the most amenable to therapeutic intervention. However, he later admitted that the 'differential diagnosis of the acquired contrary sexual feeling can be difficult'.[98] The practice in his clinic appeared to be that if a patient presented with any vestiges of heterosexual sexual feeling, they would be offered a variety of therapeutic options:

> The sexual feelings towards the other sex can be strengthened by willpower, self-control, moral, possibly hypnotic treatment, improvement of the constitution, elimination of neuroses (neurasthenia), but above all by abstinence from masturbation.[99]

Table 1.7 shows that the autobiographies in this section tended to come from younger men than the autobiographies from the other groups. Two of these men were patients in Krafft-Ebing's clinic (10.1 and 10.2)[100] but the others wrote of how they had used their own willpower (9.3),[101] regular visits to prostitutes (9.4)[102] and avoidance of masturbation (9.5)[103] to suppress their unwanted inclinations. One was a predominantly

Table 1.7 Characteristics of the men attracted to both sexes

Case study number	*Year published (repeated?)*	*Occupation*	*Age*	*Terminology*
9.1	1890 (4)	Surgeon/pathologist	31	Urning
9.2	1890 (0)	Merchant		Urning
9.3	1891 (3)	Social democrat	31	Urning, contra-sexual
9.4	1891 (2)	Official in a factory	30s	States he is not like an 'urning'
9.5	1892 (2)		31	States he is not like an 'urning'
10.1	1892 (1)		24	None
10.2	1892 (2)	Factory official	29	None

heterosexual surgeon with a foot fetish that focused on both sexes (9.1).[104] Curiously, this suicidal foot fetishist was the only one of the 'Psychic Hermaphrodites' seeking cures that was substantially repeated, published first in 1890 and then repeated four further times (9.1).[105] Although Krafft-Ebing's guiding principle when repeating autobiographies was to deploy those that were good examples, it is still striking that eight out of nine of the multiply repeated case studies came from individuals seeking neither treatment nor cure.

Neither of the men whose accounts include their clinical treatment used any word to describe their same-sex desires. Most of the other men used the word 'urning' to describe their same-sex desire, although one pointedly stated: 'I would like to comment on various statements by urnings in the published biographies that I, at least, find it very difficult to recognise as like-minded' (9.4) and another stated 'I cannot count myself in the category of so-called "urnings"' (9.5).[106] While one of the men seeking treatment had done so after a possible threat of exposure (10.2),[107] these men had mostly approached Krafft-Ebing seeking the removal of their unwanted desires in the hope of a good love marriage with a woman.

This was also a common motivation among men visiting Krafft-Ebing's clinic. In these cases, therapeutic interventions would educate the patient towards cessation of same-sex desire or sexual practice. Occasionally therapeutic intervention focused only on alleviating psychiatric comorbidities or curing addictions to masturbation. In the cases of the two autobiographers treated by Krafft-Ebing, the outcomes are not at all convincing. In the first case, the young man was willing to pay for anything that would 'cure' him but despite numerous attempts 'only a very slight degree of hypnosis, insufficient for suggestive treatment, could be achieved' (10.1).[108] The second underwent a rather more successful hypnotic therapy. His objectives were to cease masturbating, stop desiring men and desire women instead. These were only partly achieved, as he wrote to Krafft-Ebing several months later: 'From onanism I am completely cured and manly love finds no favour with me. However, full potency does not yet seem to have returned' (10.2).[109] Among the non-autobiographical clinical case studies, there were one or two that demonstrated slightly better outcomes. However, Krafft-Ebing presented what he considered his therapeutic 'successes' with very little long-term follow up, and it could have been that some patients reported positive outcomes to close off a costly therapeutic process.

1.3 Conclusion

Psychopathia Sexualis is taken by many to be the foundational text in sexology, and Krafft-Ebing's deployment of sexual autobiographies as case studies set a precedent that would shape casuistic practice in the new discipline. By tolerating and republishing case studies from urnings who did not endorse the pathologising conclusions driven by degeneration theory, Krafft-Ebing facilitated a platform of quasi-debate where urning men could self-consciously intervene in their own scientific representation. This ambivalent practice of allowing two contradictory discourses on homosexuality to sit side by side was the hallmark of *Psychopathia Sexualis* under Krafft-Ebing's editorship. It also meant that he was widely perceived by contemporary urnings as a strong ally in the fight for reform. The contemporary urning writer Otto de Joux, for instance, wrote in 1893 about a 'large Urning Association' in Germany, led by 'a famous actor',[110] which had composed a letter of heartfelt thanks to Krafft-Ebing:

> It is our sacred duty to give spontaneous expression to our gratitude for that excellent man (Dr von Krafft-Ebing) who stimulated the question of our social salvation, that noble researcher who has at last raised the Urning question in our gloomy times, so that we may strive courageously forward on the thorny path that leads to the final equality of all, and a lifting of the undeserved law that is destroying us.[111]

The high esteem in which Krafft-Ebing was held by his urning collaborators and the positive view of his casuistic practice of deploying urning autobiographies was not widely shared by some in the contemporary medical establishment. The phenomenon of urnings following the works of Krafft-Ebing and then being inspired to write to him themselves was remarked upon by a critic from forensic medicine:

> Each of the unfortunates who suffer from sexual anomalies is in the habit of following the corresponding literature with attention arbitrarily or involuntarily modelling his own history after the views he finds there, especially if they make him appear morally justified and a scientifically interesting personality.[112]

This was probably quite close to the truth in some cases. Harry Oosterhuis, who studied the original letter case studies even found one autobiography, from a Latvian nobleman called Von R., that had been structured and annotated to resemble the narrative and formal structure of a Krafft-Ebing case study.[113] Many of the other correspondents seemed to follow the general pattern of Krafft-Ebing's clinical case studies, though there is a possibility that Krafft-Ebing may have rearranged some of the contributions to fit an ordered template of content.[114] However, the same forensic medical critic did not view this practice sanguinely:

> Since the scientific works on this subject have become known to the public, it has actually come about that a large number of pederasts have found in this an excuse for their aberration. They found themselves worthy to occupy the attention of scholars and physicians. With remarkable unobjectionability they considered themselves obliged to let us in on their most secret feelings, without giving us the most repulsive details. At the same time their story is of mostly deplorable triviality.[115]

It was with criticisms like this very much in mind that the two editors who took over from Krafft-Ebing, Anton Stichl and Hugo Gugl, the directors of the Mariagrün sanatorium, addressed the phenomenon of autobiography in the 1903 edition of *Psychopathia Sexualis*: 'Autobiographies in particular have been warned against and pretty much denied all value. A truly knowledgeable person will soon recognise exaggeration and lies.'[116] Gugl and Stichl were careful to make a distinction between those seeking treatment and the rest:

> Furthermore, with those who are facing a judicial investigation, or who are forced to marriage by circumstances and rightly doubt their potency. Such people have an urgent interest in confessing the truth, in contrast to those effeminates who, moreover, are not infrequently ethically and intellectually inferior and would like to enrich science with their 'interesting medical history'.[117]

Krafft-Ebing did not share that assessment. His close alignment with his urning correspondents was not just a matter of doctor–patient empathy. His keen legal sense meant that he shared with them a deep commitment to legal reform. Over the course of his career, Krafft-Ebing did become much more outspoken in his opposition to the antisodomy laws in both Austria and Germany. In 1894 he published a thought piece on sexual law reform in which he proposed decriminalising homosexuality with an age of consent set at 18.[118] Prior to that, on 24 May 1894, Krafft-Ebing sent the manuscript to Karl Heinrich Ulrichs.[119] Ulrichs had retired to Italy several years previously and was living in Aquila writing and publishing a Latin newspaper, *Alaudae*. Krafft-Ebing's publication was an argument for the abolition of the Austrian antisodomy law, illustrated with fifty summarised urning case studies. Ulrichs devoted a large section of the July 1894 edition of *Alaudae* to a review of the manuscript.[120] By then in his final months of life, Ulrichs was so enthusiastic about this manuscript that he used it as the basis for a petition to the Austrian authorities in the last known letter he wrote.[121]

Krafft-Ebing's deployment of the autobiographical voices of same-sex attracted men and women was an avenue for them to assert their own agency, even if it was overwritten by psychiatric discourse. In one of the last things he wrote, Krafft-Ebing addressed the impact his contact with his urning patients as well as the autobiographies had made on his own scientific views. Krafft-Ebing concluded that although it was an abnormality and possibly the result of degenerative processes, homosexuality was not, after all, a pathological phenomenon. He published this paper in Magnus Hirschfeld's *Jahrbuch für sexuelle Zwischenstufen*, a sexological publication, and his conclusions perhaps reflected his deference to the editor. Krafft-Ebing acknowledged that 'contrary sexual sensation in and of itself is not a disease, but only an anomaly',[122] and that

> [i]n this way, scientific knowledge comes closer to the point of view of the contrary sexual people themselves, who never tire of emphasising, in contrast to the views of researchers, that their peculiar sexual sensation is indeed in contradiction with that of the vast majority of their sexual comrades and does not correspond to the purposes of nature, but nevertheless presents itself to them in their consciousness as an adequate, natural and thus justified one.[123]

In this, his last published work, Krafft-Ebing acknowledged that his patients and autobiographical correspondents had influenced his views. He died the next year on 22 December 1902, in Graz. For those of his correspondents who were still reading the literature, it may have come as a reassurance that their autobiographical efforts had not been in vain. His active engagement with their self-expression elevated the sexual being from the realms of smut and triviality, making their psychology an important locus of scientific study. By that time, the field of sexology was expanding on a platform where clinicians no longer saw homosexuality as the result of degenerative processes or disease. *Psychopathia Sexualis* was the foundational text in this new sexual discipline, and it set the empathetic tone for the scientists such as Albert Moll, Magnus Hirschfeld, Iwan Bloch and August Forel who would follow in his steps.

Notes

1. 'Als Verbrechen werden auch nachstehende Arten der Unzucht bestraft: I. Unzucht wider die Natur, das ist a) mit Thieren; b) mit Personen desselben Geschlechts.' (The following types of fornication are also punished as crimes: I. Fornication against nature, that is a) with animals; b) with persons of the same sex.) *Allgemeines Reichs-Gesetz- und Regierungsblatt für das Kaiserthum Österreich* 1852.
2. 'Die widernatürliche Unzucht, welche zwischen Personen männlichen Geschlechts oder von Menschen mit Thieren begangen wird, ist mit Gefängniß zu bestrafen; auch kann auf Verlust der bürgerlichen Ehrenrechte erkannt werden.' (Unnatural fornication committed between persons of the male sex or by humans with animals shall be punished by imprisonment; loss of civil rights may also be imposed.) §175 StGB, *Strafgesetzbuch für das Deutsche Reich* vom 15. Mai 1871.
3. Jens Dobler, *Zwischen Duldungspolitik und Verbrechensbekämpfung: Homosexuellenverfolgung durch die Berliner Polizei von 1848 bis 1933* (Berlin: Verlag für Polizeiwissenschaft, 2008), 208.
4. Johann Ludwig Casper, *Klinische Novellen zur gerichtlichen Medicin: nach eigenen Erfahrungen* (Berlin: Hirschwald, 1863), 36–39; Dr Scholz, 'Bekenntnisse eines an perverser Geschlechtsrichtung Leidenden', *Vierteljahrschrift für Gerichtliche Medizin* 19 (1873): 321–28.
5. Harry Oosterhuis, *Stepchildren of Nature: Krafft-Ebing, Psychiatry, and the Making of Sexual Identity* (Chicago: University of Chicago Press, 2000), 77.
6. Edward Shorter, A History of Psychiatry: From the Era of the Asylum to the Age of Prozac (New York: Wiley, 1997), 76.
7. The word 'pederast' in Germany at this time referred specifically to the crime of sodomy and had no connotations of age disparity.
8. Richard von Krafft-Ebing, 'Die Sinnestäusdungen und ihre Bedeutung für die gerichtliche Psychologie', *Friedreichs Blätter für gerichtliche Medicin*, 15/4 (1864): 243–77.
9. Oosterhuis, *Stepchildren of Nature*, 77–78.
10. 'Erst da wo die Nechtspflege den Resultaten des Naturforschers nicht mehr die Shüren vers schloß, um als bloßer Würgeengel mit dem Flammenschwert zu erscheinen, konnte die endlose Reihe der Justizmorde, Hexens prozesse und Verfolgungen ihr Ende finden.' Krafft-Ebing, 'Die Sinnestauschungen', 244, my translation.

11. Karl Heinrich Ulrichs, *Vindicta*. Leipzig: H. Matthes, 1865. Translated by Michael Lombardi-Nash as 'Book Three: Vindicta' in *The Riddle of 'Man-Manly' Love: The Pioneering Work on Male Homosexuality*, vol. 1 (Buffalo: Prometheus Books, 1994), 124.
12. They would sustain a correspondence from that point on until at least 1894, a year before Ulrichs died in exile in Italy.
13. Wilhelm Griesinger, 'Vortrag zur Eröffnung der psychiatrischen Clinik zu Berlin', *Archiv für Psychiatrie und Nervenkrankheiten* 1 (1868): 651.
14. Berliner Medicinische-Psychologische Gesellschaft 15 December 1868, *Archiv für Psychiatrie und Nervenkrankheiten* 2 (1869): 226–27.
15. Carl Friedrich Otto Westphal, 'Die conträre Sexualempfindung: Symptom eines neuropathischen (psychopathischen) Zustandes', *Archiv für Psychiatrie und Nervenkrankheiten* 2 (1869): 73–108.
16. Michel Foucault, *The History of Sexuality, Volume 1: An Introduction*, trans. Robert Hurley (New York: Vantage Books, 1990), 43.
17. Dr Schmincke, 'Ein Fall von conträrer Sexualempfindung', *Archiv für Psychiatrie und Nervenkrankheiten* 3 (1872): 225–26; Dr Scholz, 'Bekenntnisse eines an perverser Geschlechtsrichtung Leidenden', *Vierteljahrschrift für Gerichtliche Medizin* 19 (1873): 321–28; Dr H. Gock, 'Beitrag zur Kenntniss der conträren Sexualempfindung', *Archiv für Psychiatrie und Nervenkrankheiten* 5 (1875): 564–74; Dr F. Servaes, 'Zur Kenntniss von der conträren Sexualempfindung', *Archiv für Psychiatrie und Nervenkrankheiten* 6 (1876): 484–95; Siegfried Rabow, 'Über angeborene conträre Sexualempfindung', *Zeitschrift für klinische Medicin* 17 (1890): 129–43.
18. For example, Arrigo Tamassia, 'Sull'inversione dell'istinto sessuale', *Rivista sperimentale di freniatria e di medicina legale* 2 (1878): 97–117; Johan A. Backman, 'Ett fall af konträr sexualkänsla', *Finska Läkaresällskapets Handlingar* 24 (1882): 151–60; G. Alder Blumer, 'A Case of Perverted Sexual Instinct (Conträre Sexualempfindung)', *American Journal of Insanity* 39 (1882): 22–35; J. C. Shaw and G. N. Ferris, 'Perverted Sexual Instinct', *Journal of Nervous and Mental Disease* 10 (1883): 185–204; James G. Kiernan, 'Insanity: Lecture XXVI–Sexual Perversion', *Detroit Lancet* 7 (1884): 481–84; George F. Shrady, 'Perverted Sexual Instinct', *Medical Record* 26 (1884): 70–1; Julius Krueg, 'Perverted Sexual Instincts', *Brain* 4 (1881): 368–76; George Savage, 'Case of Sexual Perversion in a Man', *Journal of Mental Science* 30, no. 131 (1884): 390–91.
19. Letter from Dr Erman, a forensic physician in Hamburg, to Ulrichs, 8 February 1879. Karl Heinrich Ulrichs, *Critische Pfeile*. Leipzig: Otto und Kadler, 1880. Trans. Lombardi-Nash as 'Book Twelve: Critical Arrows' in *The Riddle of 'Man-Manly' Love,* vol. 2, §125, 686. Letter 215 in Douglas Pretsell, *The Correspondence of Karl Heinrich Ulrichs, 1846–1894* (Cham: Palgrave Macmillan, 2020), 248.

20. Richard von Krafft-Ebing, 'Ueber gewisse Anomalien des Geschlechtstriebs und die klinisch-forensische Verwerthung derselben als eines wahrscheinlich functionellen Degenerationszeichens des centralen Nervensystems', *Archiv für Psychiatrie und Nervenkrankheiten* 7 (1877): 291–312.
21. Letter from Richard von Krafft-Ebing, Graz, to Ulrichs, 29 January 1879. Ulrichs, *Critische Pfeile*, vol. 2, §125, 685. Letter 214 in Pretsell, *Correspondence*, 247.
22. 'Die conträre Sexualempfindung, wo sie angeboren vorkommt, als Theilerscheinung eines neuropsychopathischen, meist hereditären Zustands klinisch zu betrachten ist und die Bedeutung eines functionellen Degenerationszeichens hat.' Krafft-Ebing, 'Ueber gewisse Anomalien', 309, my translation.
23. Ulrichs provides his evaluation of the 'Scientific Countermovement' in an Appendix to his final work. Ulrichs, *Critische Pfeile*, §125–26, 685–88.
24. Ulrichs, *Critische Pfeile*, 685.
25. Ulrichs, *Critische Pfeile*, 688.
26. Oosterhuis, *Stepchildren of Nature*, 79–81.
27. Oosterhuis, *Stepchildren of Nature*, 85.
28. Oosterhuis, *Stepchildren of Nature*, 91.
29. Oosterhuis, *Stepchildren of Nature*, 94.
30. Richard von Krafft-Ebing, 'Zur "conträren Sexualempfindung" in klinisch-forensischer Hinsicht', *Allgemeine Zeitschrift für Psychiatrie* 38 (1882): 211–27.
31. Neurasthenia was a loosely defined minor psychiatric definition very much of the time period with a collection of symptoms including headache, lethargy, tiredness and irritability.
32. Krafft-Ebing, 'Zur "conträren Sexualempfindung"', 213.
33. Krafft-Ebing, 'Zur "conträren Sexualempfindung"', 215–16.
34. Krafft-Ebing, 'Zur "conträren Sexualempfindung"', 216.
35. Krafft-Ebing, 'Zur "conträren Sexualempfindung"', 222.
36. In each case where an autobiography is referred to within this introduction, it will be indicated with the bracketed number.
37. Richard von Krafft-Ebing, *Lehrbuch der Psychiatrie auf klinischer Grundlage für practische Ärzte und Studirende*, 2nd ed. (Stuttgart: Ferdinand Enke, 1883), 85–88.
38. Krafft-Ebing, *Lehrbuch*, 85–88; Richard von Krafft-Ebing, 'Zur Lehre von der conträren Sexualempfindung', *Der Irrenfreund* 26 (1884): 1–14; Richard von Krafft-Ebing, 'Die conträre Sexualempfindung vor dem Forum', *Jahrbücher für Psychiatrie* 6 (1885): 34–47.
39. After Krafft-Ebing's death, *Psychopathia Sexualis* continued to be updated under a succession of different editors up to the seventeenth edition in 1924, edited by Albert Moll.

40. Richard von Krafft-Ebing, *Neue Forschungen auf dem Gebiet der Psychopathia Sexualis: Eine medicinisch-psychologische Studie* (Stuttgart: Ferdinand Enke, 1890); Richard von Krafft-Ebing, *Neue Forschungen auf dem Gebiet der Psychopathia Sexualis: Eine medicinisch-psychologische Studie* (Stuttgart: Ferdinand Enke, 1891); Richard von Krafft-Ebing, 'Neue Forschungen auf dem Gebiet der Psychopathia Sexualis', *Jahrbuch für sexuelle Zwischenstufen* 3 (1901): 1–36.
41. Richard von Krafft-Ebing, 'Zur conträren Sexualempfindung: Autobiographie und strafrechtliche Betrachtungen über den Paragraphen 175 des deutschen Strafgesetzbuchs von einem Conträr-Sexualen', *Friedreichs Blätter für gerichtliche Medicin* 42 (1891): 385–400; Richard von Krafft-Ebing, 'Zur conträren Sexualempfindung: Autobiographie und strafrechtliche Betrachtungen von einem conträr Sexualen', *Wiener medizinische Blätter* 15 (1892): 42–44.
42. This is not a complete table of all Krafft-Ebing's works in this period. He wrote several other works on different subjects not included here. These are the papers and books (including editions 1–11 of *Psychopathia Sexualis*) that include all of the case studies of same-sex attracted and gender nonconforming men and women.
43. The four categories Krafft-Ebing used were as follows: (1) *Psychische Hermaphrodisie* (Psychic Hermaphrodites); (2) *Homosexuale oder Urninge* (Homosexuals or Urnings); (3) *Effeminatio und Viraginität* (Effeminates and Viragines); (4) *Androgyne und Gynandrier* (Androgynes and Gynandres). Richard von Krafft-Ebing, *Psychopathia Sexualis: Mit besonderer Berücksichtigung der conträren Sexualempfindung. Eine klinisch-forensische Studie*, 4th ed. (Stuttgart: Ferdinand Enke, 1889), 96–183.
44. In Austria, in particular, the authorities tended to take a pragmatic attitude to prostitution. The thinking was that criminalising prostitution did not reduce its occurrence and that if lower-class women could provide a sexual outlet for bourgeois men that would in some way protect bourgeois women from sexual violence. In Vienna prostitution was legal with prostitutes registered to the police and required to supply medical certificates twice per week. Elsewhere in Austria a variety of local statutes regulated prostitution to various degrees. In Germany, prostitution was tacitly legal, but attitudes to sex work were ambivalent. Ostensibly, the German legal code of 1871 banned brothels and the commercial availability of sex, but this was relaxed in 1876 to apply only to sex workers not regulated by the police.
45. Richard von Krafft-Ebing, *Psychopathia Sexualis: Mit besonderer Berücksichtigung der conträren Sexualempfindung. Eine klinisch-forensische Studie*, 5th ed. (Stuttgart: Ferdinand Enke, 1890), 174.

46. Harry Oosterhuis, who had access to the original letters stated that the 'unpublished case histories are in no way different from the published ones'. It appears, then, that Krafft-Ebing did not substantially edit the letter autobiographies he published. Oosterhuis, *Stepchildren of Nature*, 195.
47. Krafft-Ebing, *Irrenfreund* 26 (1884): 2–14.
48. Richard von Krafft-Ebing, 'Die conträre Sexualempfindung vor dem Forum', *Jahrbücher für Psychiatrie* 6 (1885): 34–47.
49. 'Die Liebe zu Männern kann ich nicht krankhaft finden. Ich würde mich daher psychisch vollkommen gesund halten, wenn mich nicht in meinem Geschlechtsleben eine sonderbare Manie verfolgen und peinigen würde.' Krafft-Ebing, 'Die conträre Sexualempfindung', 42, my translation.
50. 'Wann wird man anfangen, auch im grossem Publicum der Sache ohne Vorurtheil näher zu treten? Die Wissenschaft darf jedenfalls keinen Augenblick innehalten, die gewonnenen Resultate möglichst zu verbreiten und auch dem Laien verständlich zu machen.' Krafft-Ebing, 'Die conträre Sexualempfindung', 42, my translation.
51. 'Erst als ich etwa 30 Jahre war, kamen mir die Schriften von Numa (Ulrichs) in die Hand und ich kann nicht schildern, welche Erlösung es für mich war, zu erfahren, dass es noch viele andere Männer gebe, die gerade so geschlechtlich beanlagt sind, wie ich selbst, und dass das, was ich geschlechtlich empfand, keine Verirrung, sondern eine mir von der Natur innewohnende besondere geschlechtliche Anlage sei, Ich öffnete die Augen und fand bald in meiner nächsten Nähe gleichgestimmte Naturen. Zum erstenmale nun erfuhr ich den Genuss, durch directe Berührung eines Manneskörpers die geschlechtliche Befriedigung zu finden. Ich suchte nicht mehr in vergeblicher Weise gegen eine mir tief eingepflanzte Veranlagung anzukämpfen.' Krafft-Ebing, 'Die conträre Sexualempfindung', 46, my translation.
52. '[S]eit ich meiner urningischen Natur mehr freien Lauf lasse, bin ich glücklicher, gesunder und leistungsfähiger!' Krafft-Ebing, 'Die conträre Sexualempfindung', 46, my translation.
53. Krafft-Ebing, 'Die conträre Sexualempfindung', 36.
54. Krafft-Ebing, *Psychopathia Sexualis*, 5th ed., 170–75.
55. Krafft-Ebing, *Psychopathia Sexualis*, 5th ed., 170–75.
56. Krafft-Ebing, *Psychopathia Sexualis*, 4th ed., 216–9.
57. Krafft-Ebing described the author of this letter as 'a highly placed man in London'. Symonds was at the time living in Davos, Switzerland. The authorship of this letter came to light after Symonds's death when the manuscript was discovered with his memoirs. It was passed to Edith Lees, wife of Havelock Ellis, who transcribed it. Sean Brady, *John Addington Symonds (1840–1893) and Homosexuality: A Critical Edition of Sources* (London: Palgrave Macmillan, 2012), 209.

58. Krafft-Ebing, 'Zur conträren Sexualempfindung', *Friedreichs Blätter* (1891): 385–400.
59. Richard von Krafft-Ebing, *Psychopathia Sexualis: Eine klinisch-forensische Studie*, 1st ed. (Stuttgart: Ferdinand Enke, 1886), 64–68.
60. Richard von Krafft-Ebing, *Psychopathia Sexualis. Mit besonderer Berücksichtigung der conträren Sexualempfindung: Eine klinisch-forensische Studie,* 3rd ed. (Stuttgart: Ferdinand Enke, 1888), 87–91.
61. Richard von Krafft-Ebing, *Psychopathia Sexualis. Mit besonderer Berücksichtigung der conträren Sexualempfindung: Eine klinisch-forensische Studie,* 2nd ed. (Stuttgart: Ferdinand Enke, 1887), 80–85.
62. Krafft-Ebing, *Psychopathia Sexualis*, 2nd ed., 85–91.
63. Krafft-Ebing, *Neue Forschungen* (1891), 130.
64. Krafft-Ebing, *Neue Forschungen* (1890), 46.
65. Oosterhuis, *Stepchildren of Nature*, 164.
66. Krafft-Ebing, *Psychopathia Sexualis*, 5th ed., 161.
67. Krafft-Ebing, *Psychopathia Sexualis*, 5th ed., 158.
68. Oosterhuis, *Stepchildren of Nature*, 206.
69. The four case studies of women that Henry Havelock Ellis and John Addington Symonds deployed in *Sexual Inversion* were all voluntarily submitted as sexual autobiographies by friends of Ellis's wife Edith Lees. Although these women were English and their biographies were paraphrased rather than quoted from, the first edition of this book was published in Germany in 1896: Henry Havelock Ellis and John Addington Symonds, *Das konträre Geschlechtsgefühl* (Leipzig: G. H. Wigand, 1896).
70. Richard von Krafft-Ebing, *Psychopathia Sexualis: Mit besonderer Berücksichtigung der conträren Sexualempfindung. Eine klinisch-forensische Studie,* 10th ed. (Stuttgart: Ferdinand Enke, 1898), 254.
71. Krafft-Ebing, *Psychopathia Sexualis*, 4th ed., 173–74.
72. Richard von Krafft-Ebing, *Psychopathia Sexualis: Mit besonderer Berücksichtigung der conträren Sexualempfindung: Eine klinisch-forensische Studie,* 9th ed. (Stuttgart: Ferdinand Enke, 1894), 285–8.
73. Krafft-Ebing, *Psychopathia Sexualis*, 4th ed., 76–77, 173–74.
74. Krafft-Ebing, *Psychopathia Sexualis*, 4th ed., 76.
75. Krafft-Ebing, *Psychopathia Sexualis*, 10th ed., 264.
76. Krafft-Ebing, *Psychopathia Sexualis*, 9th ed., 285–88.
77. Krafft-Ebing, *Psychopathia Sexualis*, 10th ed., 263–64.
78. Krafft-Ebing, *Psychopathia Sexualis*, 4th ed., 76–77.
79. Krafft-Ebing, *Psychopathia Sexualis*, 4th ed., 173–74
80. Krafft-Ebing, *Psychopathia Sexualis*, 4th ed., 180.
81. Krafft-Ebing, 'Neue Forschungen' (1901): 30–1.
82. Oosterhuis, *Stepchildren of Nature*, 251.
83. Krafft-Ebing, *Psychopathia Sexualis*, 5th ed., 213–20.
84. Krafft-Ebing, *Psychopathia Sexualis*, 5th ed., 219.

85. Krafft-Ebing, *Neue Forschungen* (1890), 63–66.
86. Krafft-Ebing, *Neue Forschungen* (1890), 66–79.
87. Katie Sutton, '"We Too Deserve a Place in the Sun": The Politics of Transvestite Identity in Weimar Germany', *German Studies Review* 35/2 (2012): 337–38.
88. Richard Ekins and Dave King, *The Transgender Phenomenon* (New York: SAGE Publications, 2006), 61–64.
89. Richard von Krafft-Ebing, *Psychopathia Sexualis: Mit besonderer Berücksichtigung der conträren Sexualempfindung: Eine klinisch-forensische Studie,* 3rd ed. (Stuttgart: Ferdinand Enke, 1888), 77–80; Krafft-Ebing, *Psychopathia Sexualis*, 4th ed., 131–38; Krafft-Ebing, *Neue Forschungen* (1891), 123–27.
90. 'N. N, ein durchaus objectiver, ruhiger Herr, meinte zu X: "Wenn wir doch wenigstens es durchsetzen könnten, dass man die conträre Sexualempfindung für pathologisch ansieht, dass wir nicht mehr für Verbrecher gehalten werden." X entgegnete darauf: "Niemals kann ich dem beistimmen; lieber wähle ich noch den heutigen Zustand. Wir werden von den anderen doch nur majorisirt, und wenn man die Affection für krankhaft ansieht, dann steckt man uns ins Irrenhaus."' Albert Moll, *Die Conträre Sexualempfindung, Mit Benutzung amtlichen Materials* (Berlin: Fischer, 1891), 75n.
91. 'Die von Tarnowsky (op. cit. p. 17 u. flP.) behauptete Möglichkeit, dass ein wirklicher, mit angeborener Perversion des Sexuallebens behafteter Urning durch Erziehung von seiner krankhaften Geschlechtsrichtung befreit und zu normaler Geschlechtsempfindung gebracht werden könne, muss ich auf Grund meiner Erfahrungen verneinen.' Krafft-Ebing, *Psychopathia Sexualis*, 1st ed., 64, my translation.
92. Krafft-Ebing, *Psychopathia Sexualis*, 3rd ed., 94; Krafft-Ebing, *Psychopathia Sexualis*, 5th ed., 115.
93. Krafft-Ebing, *Psychopathia Sexualis*, 3rd ed., 93; Krafft-Ebing, *Psychopathia Sexualis*, 4th ed., 138.
94. Krafft-Ebing, *Psychopathia Sexualis*, 5th ed., 117; Krafft-Ebing, *Neue Forschungen* (1891), 102.
95. Krafft-Ebing, *Psychopathia Sexualis*, 3rd ed., 92.
96. Krafft-Ebing, *Neue Forschungen* (1891), 125.
97. 'Bei (angeborener) psychischer Hermaphrodisie debütirt die Vita sexualis immer im Sinne der homosexualen weit stärker veranlagten Richtung, bei erworbener conträrer Sexualempfindung ist das Debüt im heterosexualen Sinne und die homosexuale Richtung tritt auf und entwickelt sich auf Grund greifbarer Gelegenheitsursachen' (masturbatorische Neurasthenie, psychische Momente).' Krafft-Ebing, *Psychopathia Sexualis*, 4th ed., 97, my translation.

98. 'Schwierig kann die differentielle Diagnose von der erworbenen conträren Sexualempfindung sein.' Krafft-Ebing, *Psychopathia Sexualis*, 9th ed., 244, my translation.
99. 'Die sexuellen Empfindungen gegenüber dem anderen Greschlecht können durch Willenskraft, Selbstzucht, moralische, ev. hypnotische Behandlung, Besserung der Constitution, Beseitigung von Neurosen (Neurasthenie), vor Allem aber durch Abstinenz von Masturbation gekräftigt werden.' Krafft-Ebing, *Psychopathia Sexualis*, 4th ed., 96, my translation.
100. Richard von Krafft-Ebing, *Psychopathia Sexualis: Mit besonderer Berücksichtigung der conträren Sexualempfindung: Eine klinisch-forensische Studie,* 7th ed. (Stuttgart: Ferdinand Enke, 1892), 241–45; Krafft-Ebing, Psychopathia Sexualis, 7th ed., 326–29.
101. Richard von Krafft-Ebing, *Psychopathia Sexualis: Mit besonderer Berücksichtigung der conträren Sexualempfindung: Eine klinisch-forensische Studie,* 6th ed. (Stuttgart: Ferdinand Enke, 1891), 240.
102. Krafft-Ebing, *Neue Forschungen* (1891), 105.
103. Krafft-Ebing, *Psychopathia Sexualis*, 7th ed., 196.
104. Krafft-Ebing, *Psychopathia Sexualis*, 5th ed., 110–13.
105. Krafft-Ebing, *Psychopathia Sexualis*, 5th ed., 110–13.
106. Krafft-Ebing, *Neue Forschungen* (1891), 109–110; Krafft-Ebing, *Psychopathia Sexualis*, 7th ed., 197.
107. Krafft-Ebing, *Psychopathia Sexualis*, 7th ed., 327.
108. Krafft-Ebing, *Psychopathia Sexualis*, 7th ed., 245.
109. Krafft-Ebing, *Psychopathia Sexualis*, 7th ed., 329.
110. De Joux does not mention the actor's name, but it was possibly Josef Gottfried Ignaz Kainz. Kainz, an Austrian, had been performing on the Berlin stage since 1883 and was one of Germany's most famous actors. Dazzlingly handsome, he had been a close favourite and possible lover of Ludwig II. Though married, Kainz was bisexual, and in Berlin, he maintained a salon of young attractive artists and poets. Bernd-Ulrich Hergemöller, ed., *Mann für Mann: Biographisches Lexikon zur Geschichte von Freundesliebe und mannmännlicher Sexualität im deutschen Sprachraum*, vol. 1 (A-RAS) (Berlin: LIT, 2010), 619–21.
111. 'Es ist uns heilige Pflicht, unserer Dankbarkeit für jenen ausgezeichneten Mann (Dr von Krafft-Ebing.) spontanen Ausdruck zu geben, welcher die Frage unserer gesellschaftlichen Rettung angeregt, jenem edlen Forscher, welcher endlich die Urningfrage aufgerollt hat in unserer düsteren Zeit, aus daß wir mutig vorwärts streben auf dem dornenvollen Pfade, der zur endlichen Gleichberechtigung Aller, und einer Aufhebung des unverdienten Bannes führt, welcher uns vernichtet.' Otto de Joux, *Die Enterbten des Liebesglückes, oder Das dritte Geschlecht.* Leipzig: Spohr, 1893, 73, my translation.

112. 'Jeder der Unglücklichen, die an geschlechtlichen Anomalien lei den, pflegt die entsprechende Literatur mit Aufmerksamkeit zu verfolgen, willkürlich oder unwillkürlich modelt er seine eigene Geschichte nach den Ansichten, die er dort findet, besonders wenn sie ihn als moralisch gerechtfertigt und als eine wissenschaftlich interessante Persönlichkeit erscheinen lassen.' Fritz Strassmann, *Lehrbuch der gerichtlichen Medizin*, Auflag 1 (Berlin: Ferdinand Enke, 1895), 122, my translation. The fuller quotation in German can be found in Klaus Müller, *Aber in meinem Herzen sprach eine Stimme so laut: Homosexuelle Autobiographien und medizinische Pathographien im neunzehnten Jahrhundert* (Berlin: rosa Winkel, 1991), 259.
113. Oosterhuis, *Stepchildren of Nature*, 2–6.
114. Douglas Pretsell, 'The Evolution of the Questionnaire in German Sexual Science: A Methodological Narrative,' *History of Science* 58, no. 3 (2020), 343.
115. 'Seit die wissenscha ft lichen Arbeiten über diesen Gegenstand im Publicum bekannt geworden sind, ist es thatsächlich dahin gekommen, dass eine grosse Zahl Päderasten hierin eine Entschuldigung ihrer Verirrung gefunden hat. Sie fanden sich würdig, die Aufmerksamkeit der Gelehrten und Aerzte zu beschäftigen. Mit bemerkenswerther Unbedenklichkeit hielten sie sich für verpflichtet, uns in ihre geheimsten Gefühle einzuweihen, ohne uns dabei die abstossendsten Details zu schenken. Dabei ist ihre Geschichte von zumeist kläglicher Trivialität.' Strassmann, *Lehrbuch*, 122, my translation. The fuller quotation in German can be found in Müller, *Aber in meinem Herzen*, 259.
116. 'Namentlich vor den Autobiographien hat man gewarnt und ihnen so ziemlich allen Werth abgesprochen. Ein wirklich Sachverstän diger wird Uebertreibung und Lüge bald erkennen.' H. Gugl and A. Stichl, *Psychopathia Sexualis. Mit besonderer Berücksichtigung der konträren Sexualempfindung. Eine medicinisch-gerichtiche Studie für Ärzte und Juristen*, 12th ed. (Stuttgart: Ferdinand Enke, 1903), 308, my translation.
117. 'ferner bei solchen, die einer gerichtlichen Unter suchung entgegensehen, oder die durch die Verhältnisse zum Hei rathen gezwungen sind und mit Recht an ihrer Potenz zweifeln. Solche haben ein dringendes Interesse, die Wahrheit zu bekennen, im Gegensatz zu jenen Effeminirten, die zudem nicht selten ethisch und intellectuell minderwerthig sind und die Wissenschaft mit ihrer "interessanten Krankengeschichte" bereichern möchten.' Gugl and Stichl, *Psychopathia Sexualis*, 12th ed., 309, my translation.
118. Richard von Krafft-Ebing, *Der Conträrsexuale vor dem Strafrichter* (Vienna: Franz Deutige, 1895).

119. None of the letters has survived (other than the one Ulrichs published himself in *Critische Pfeile*), but it seems as if the two maintained lines of communication over many years, even after Ulrichs moved to Italy.
120. Karl Heinrich Ulrichs, *Alaudae, Eine lateinische Zeitschrift, 1889–1895*, Nachdruck mit einer Einleitung von Wilfried Stroh (Hamburg: MännerschwarmSkript Verlag, 2004), 355–58.
121. Letter from Ulrichs to Members of the Austrian Royal and Imperial Ministry of Justice, 18 June 1894. Letter 227 in Pretsell, *Correspondence*, 260–62.
122. '[D]ie konträre Sexualempfindung an und für sich keine Krankheit, sondern nur eine Anomalie bedeutet.' Krafft-Ebing, 'Neue Forschungen', 2, my translation.
123. 'Damit nähert sich die wissenschaftliche Erkenntnis dem Standpunkt der konträr Sexualen selbst, die nicht müde wurden, im Gegensatz zu den Anschauungen der Forscher zu betonen, dass ihre eigenartige Geschlechtsempfindung zwar im Widerspruch mit der der übergrossen Majorität ihrer Geschlechtsgenossen sei und den Zwecken der Natur nicht entsprechend, gleichwohl in ihrem Bewusstsein als eine adaequate, natürliche und damit berechtigte sich ihnen darstelle.' Krafft-Ebing, 'Neue Forschungen', 2, my translation.

Annotation and Abbreviations

Bb	Beobachtung [case study]
R:	Repeats
LB (1883)	Richard von Krafft-Ebing, *Lehrbuch der Psychiatrie auf klinischer Grundlage für practische Ärzte und Studirende*, 2nd ed. (Stuttgart: Ferdinand Enke, 1883).
DI (1884)	Richard von Krafft-Ebing, 'Zur Lehre von der conträren Sexualempfindung', *Der Irrenfreund* 26 (1884): 1–14.
JP (1885)	Richard von Krafft-Ebing, 'Die conträre Sexualempfindung vor dem Forum', *Jarbücher für Psychiatrie* 6 (1885): 34–47.
PS1 (1886)	Richard von Krafft-Ebing, *Psychopathia Sexualis: Eine klinisch-forensische Studie* (Stuttgart: Ferdinand Enke, 1886).
PS2 (1887)	Richard von Krafft-Ebing, *Psychopathia Sexualis: Mit besonderer Berücksichtigung der conträren Sexualempfindung. Eine klinisch-forensische Studie*, 2nd ed. (Stuttgart: Ferdinand Enke, 1887).
PS3 (1888)	Richard von Krafft-Ebing, *Psychopathia Sexualis: Mit besonderer Berücksichtigung der conträren Sexualempfindung. Eine klinisch-forensische Studie*, 3rd ed. (Stuttgart: Ferdinand Enke, 1888).
PS4 (1889)	Richard von Krafft-Ebing, *Psychopathia Sexualis: Mit besonderer Berücksichtigung der conträren Sexualempfindung. Eine klinisch-forensische Studie*, 4th ed. (Stuttgart: Ferdinand Enke, 1889).
PS5 (1890)	Richard von Krafft-Ebing, *Psychopathia Sexualis: Mit besonderer Berücksichtigung der conträren Sexualempfindung. Eine klinisch-forensische Studie*, 5th ed. (Stuttgart: Ferdinand Enke, 1890).
NF (1890)	Richard von Krafft-Ebing, *Neue Forschungen auf dem Gebiet der Psychopathia Sexualis: Eine medicinisch-psychologische Studie* (Stuttgart: Ferdinand Enke, 1890).
PS6 (1891)	Richard von Krafft-Ebing, *Psychopathia Sexualis: Mit besonderer Berücksichtigung der conträren Sexualempfindung. Eine klinisch-forensische Studie*, 6th ed. (Stuttgart: Ferdinand Enke, 1891).
NF (1891)	Richard von Krafft-Ebing, *Neue Forschungen auf dem Gebiet der Psychopathia Sexualis: Eine medicinisch-psychologische Studie* (Stuttgart: Ferdinand Enke, 1891).
FB (1891)	Richard von Krafft-Ebing, 'Zur conträren Sexualempfindung: Autobiographie und strafrechtliche Betrachtungen über den §175 des deutchen Strafgesetzbuchs von einem Conträr-Sexualen', *Friedreich's Blätter für gerichtliche Medicin* 42 (1891): 385–400.

(*continued*)

(continued)

PS7 (1892)	Richard von Krafft-Ebing, *Psychopathia Sexualis: Mit besonderer Berücksichtigung der conträren Sexualempfindung. Eine klinisch-forensische Studie*, 7th ed. (Stuttgart: Ferdinand Enke, 1892).
PS8 (1893)	Richard von Krafft-Ebing, *Psychopathia Sexualis: Mit besonderer Berücksichtigung der conträren Sexualempfindung. Eine klinisch-forensische Studie*, 8th ed. (Stuttgart: Ferdinand Enke, 1893).
PS9 (1894)	Richard von Krafft-Ebing, *Psychopathia Sexualis: Mit besonderer Berücksichtigung der conträren Sexualempfindung. Eine klinisch-forensische Studie*, 9th ed. (Stuttgart: Ferdinand Enke, 1894).
PS10 (1898)	Richard von Krafft-Ebing, *Psychopathia Sexualis: Mit besonderer Berücksichtigung der conträren Sexualempfindung. Eine klinisch-forensische Studie*, 10th ed. (Stuttgart: Ferdinand Enke, 1898).
PS11 (1901)	Richard von Krafft-Ebing, *Psychopathia Sexualis: Mit besonderer Berücksichtigung der conträren Sexualempfindung. Eine klinisch-forensische Studie*, 11th ed. (Stuttgart: Ferdinand Enke, 1901).

CHAPTER 2

The First Autobiography

2.1 LB (1883) Bb 2, 85–8

R: *PS2 (1887) Bb 26, PS6 (1891) Bb 83*

[KRAFFT-EBING: Mr X., 33 years old, Hungarian by birth, wholesaler, consulted me one day because of insomnia and neurasthenic complaints he had been suffering from for years. The investigation of the causes of the complaint led to the patient's confession that he had an abnormal sexual drive towards his own sex, that he was in general very in need of sex, and that his nervous complaint probably derived from this. The patient, an intelligent man, allowed himself to be persuaded to share the story of his life and suffering, from which the following might be of scientific interest.]

My abnormal sex sensation goes back to my childhood. At the age of three, a fashion journal came into my hands. I kissed the perfectly beautiful male figures until I tore the paper; I paid no attention to the female figures. Boys' games were disgusting to me. I preferred playing with girls because there were always dolls. I loved to make dolls' clothes; I am still interested in dolls today, despite my 33 years. Even as a boy, I could spend hours on the lookout for decent places to get a glimpse of the genitals of men. If I succeeded, I came to feel very strange and dizzy. Weak, unsympathetic men or even boys were indifferent to me. At the age of 13 I surrendered to onanism. From the age of 13–15 I slept in the same bed with

D. Pretsell, *Queer Voices in the Works of Richard von Krafft-Ebing, 1883–1901*, Genders and Sexualities in History,
https://doi.org/10.1007/978-3-031-17331-8_2

a handsome young man. That was happiness! For hours in the evening I waited, erect, for him to come home. Then, when he happened to brush my genitals in bed, I had a moment of bliss. When I was 14, I had a schoolmate who felt the same way I did. For hours during class, we held each other's genitals in our hands. Oh, those were blissful hours! As often as I could, I went to the baths. That was always a feast for me. The sight of male genitals gave me violent erections. At the age of 16 I came to the big city. Seeing so many beautiful men delighted me. At the age of 17-and-a-half I tried to have intercourse with a prostitute but was unable to do so because of disgust and fear. Further attempts also failed until the age of 19. There I finally succeeded, but the sexual intercourse gave me no pleasure, rather disgust. I overcame myself and was proud of my success in still being a man, something I had gradually begun to doubt. Later attempts were unsuccessful. I now considered myself impotent, consulted doctors, visited baths and water cures to cure my supposed impotence, for I still did not know what to make of it. I liked to be in ladies' company, perhaps out of vanity, as I seemed likeable and amiable to most ladies. But I only appreciated mental aesthetic merits in ladies. I liked to dance with them, but if one of them snuggled up to me during the dance, I felt a strong aversion, even disgust, and would have liked to beat her up. If it happened that a gentleman danced with me for a joke, I was always a lady. There I pressed and snuggled up to him and was quite happy and blissful. When I was 18 years old, a gentleman who came to our café once said: 'That's a sweet boy, you could charge a pound a day for him in the Orient'. That gave me a headache. Another gentleman liked to joke with me, often robbing me of kisses on my way out, which I would have liked to give him myself. This kiss robber later came to be a lover of mine. These circumstances were noted by me, and I waited for an opportunity.

When I was about 25 years old, it happened that a former Capuchin monk took a firm hold of me. He came to me like a Mephisto. He finally spoke to me. Even today I think I can still feel the beating of my heart from that time, I was close to fainting. He invited me to a rendezvous at an inn for the evening. I went, but turned back at the threshold; I suspected dreadful horrors. The second evening the Capuchin found me again. He persuaded me and took me to his room; as I was so excited, I couldn't walk. My seducer sat me down on the couch, fixed me smiling with his wonderful black eyes, and I lost consciousness.

I would have to write too much about this lust, this idealistic, divine bliss that filled my being; I think only a boy who is head-over-heels in love, who is still completely innocent, who has been able to satisfy his longing for love for the first time can be as happy as I was that evening. My seducer demanded my life for fun (which I took seriously at first). I asked him to let me be happy for a while longer, then I would have ended my life united with him. It would have been according to my exaggerated ideas at that time. I then had a five-year relationship with the man who is still so dear to me. Oh, how happy and yet often unhappy I was at that time! If I only saw him talking to a handsome young man, a raging jealousy arose in me. At the age of 27, I became engaged to a young lady. Her spirit and fine aesthetic sense, as well as financial considerations for my business, prompted me to think of marriage with her. Moreover, I am a great lover of children, and as often as I met the most ordinary day labourer with his wife and a pretty child, I envied the man his family happiness. So I was self-satisfied and got through the time of the bride's marriage with ease, but I felt more fear and anxiety than pleasure at my bride's kisses. Once or twice, however, it happened that I got an erection through hearty kissing after a rich night's meal. How happy I was then; I already saw myself as a daddy! Twice I came close to cancelling the marriage. On the wedding day, when the guests were already gathered, I locked myself in a room, cried like a child and absolutely did not want to have the marriage. At the persuasion of all the relatives, to whom I gave the first best excuses, I was dragged from a street toilet and down the aisle.

Fortunately, my wife was having her period at the time of the wedding. Oh, how I thanked all the saints for this blessing! I am still convinced today that only this made it possible for me to have intercourse later. Why it came to be possible for me to later join my wife and have a hearty boy, I do not know. He is my consolation in my life, which has been so misguided. I can only thank God for the good fortune of having a child. I swindled my way, so to speak, in the marriage bed. My wife, whom I hold in high esteem because of her excellent qualities, has no idea of my condition, only that she complains: often about my coldness. With her kindness of heart and naivety, it was possible for me to make her believe that the performance of marital duty occurs only once a month. Since she is not very sensual and, moreover, I find an excuse in my nervousness, I manage to swindle my way through. Coitus is my greatest sacrifice. By drinking copious amounts of wine and using erections that occur in the morning when my bladder is full, I manage to perform it about once a month, but I have no feeling of lust, I feel completely dull, and my nervous complaints increase for days. Only the consciousness of the fulfilled marital duty, towards the otherwise beloved wife, is then moral success and satisfaction for me. With a man, it is different. I can attend him several times during the night, feeling myself in the sexual role of the man. I feel the highest lust, the purest happiness, and feel refreshed and delighted by it. In more recent times, my urge for men has diminished somewhat. I even have the courage to avoid a beautiful young man who shows interest in me. Will it come to last? I fear not. I absolutely cannot be without male love, and when I must do without it, I am depressed, feel dull, miserable, have pain and pressure in my head. I have always felt that my remarkable eccentricity is something innate and pathological, but I would feel happy if only I were not married. My good wife takes care of me. Often, I am gripped by the fear that I can't stand it with her any longer. Then thoughts come to me of divorcing her, killing myself, escaping to America.

CHAPTER 3

Dissenters

3.1 DI (1884) Bb 1, 2–5

R: *PS4 (1889) Bb 71, PS6 (1891) Bb 94*

I read your work in the *Zeitschrift für Psychiatrie*. I am redeemed by it, and certainly thousands with me, in the eyes of every thinking and semi-honest person, and I thank you most warmly for it. You know yourself how much our cause comes to be frowned upon, despised and persecuted. I can well understand why scientific research is so late in taking up this phenomenon—it remains a disgusting unnatural crime in the eyes of a sane person who is not familiar with it. I believe that Ulrichs still underestimates the frequency of its occurrence. In my hometown (18,000 inhabitants), I know 14 urnings personally. In a city of 60,000 inhabitants, I know at least 80.

If I may be so free to take up your time with a small curriculum vitae, I will proceed with all openness. Perhaps this will provide you with further clues for a critical assessment of the way of urnings. You may dispose of these remarks as you see fit, even if not under my name.

Music and literature have always been my hobbyhorses. My whole disposition is feminine; I hate all noise, ribaldry and discord. As a child, I always hung around with the girls, always took part in their games with dolls and cooking utensils, liked to dress up in female finery, which is why

D. Pretsell, *Queer Voices in the Works of Richard von Krafft-Ebing, 1883–1901*, Genders and Sexualities in History,
https://doi.org/10.1007/978-3-031-17331-8_3

I was also called the girls' clown. Even though I later took part in gymnastics and drill as a schoolboy, my greatest pleasure was helping my mother with her household chores. Around the age of 13, I reached maturity, that is, the sexual attraction to another being, but a male one. At school I always had my lover and came to be terribly jealous of girls or other schoolmates who were preferred by my darling over me. Kissing him was my pleasure, a sexual touch overcame my sense of propriety, although it was the goal of my desires. You will be surprised to learn that until the age of 28 I never had a seminal discharge, neither through pollutions, nor through onanism, nor through a sexual act with a man.

As a young man, I had a serious love affair with a student. He did reciprocate my love, but only in the true rapturous friendship of youth, for when we once happened to sleep together and my member became understandably excited, he quite naively asked me if I thought he was a girl. I was only allowed to kiss him, and he returned my kisses. We raved about poetry, literature, beautiful things, as was usual in those years. Saying goodbye to him was an almost heart-breaking experience for me. The young girls in my headmaster's house left me cold. I was on friendly terms with them in a completely unbiased way. New, thoroughly platonic love affairs with young men followed; but despite the most pleasant external circumstances, I was often overcome by the depressing feeling—you are not like the others, and this always occurred most depressingly when I was in the company of merry comrades who were boasting in the fresh exuberance of life, even cracking jokes. I didn't know whether to laugh or cry. This was an unpleasant state of affairs; I was forced to operate against my nature, to throw sand in the eyes of others. In God's name, I can only get rid of this dilemma in the company of like-minded people. It is therefore natural to seek them out, even if it might have been wiser to avoid them. In the company of beautiful young ladies, I have never felt the immediate tension of the mental powers that develop to please—but I have felt it in the presence of charming men. I also prefer to associate with married women or with very naive young ladies—any intention to lure me into the marriage yarn upsets me, and I am sensitive to the point of stupidity on this point.

Until I was 28, I had no idea that others besides myself were like me. One evening, in the castle square in X, where, as I later noticed, the urnings are wont to seek and find each other, I met a man who aroused me sexually so much that semen was ejaculated. Of course, this meant that I lost the person who had been my best friend until then, because I now often went to the castle square and later sought out such places in other larger cities. Nevertheless, you will believe me that this realisation also brought me a certain comfort—I would like to say the comfort of belonging together and of not being alone, and that the depressing feeling that I did not really belong to human society was taken away. The love affairs that followed at least gave my life a certain charm that I had never known before. But I was hurrying towards my doom. I had established an intimate relationship with a young man. He was extremely eccentric, romantic, amorous, easy-going and penniless. He took me completely in his hand, considered himself my legal spouse. I had to take him into the shop with me. Hardly believable scenes of jealousy now took place in my house. He repeatedly attempted suicide by poisoning himself and I saved his life with great difficulty. I suffered terribly from his jealousy, tyranny, bossiness and arrogance. He beat me in his jealousy, threatened to reveal my secret to the courts. I always had to be aware of this eventuality. Repeatedly, it took great sacrifices of money to get this obviously insane lover out of the house. His passion for me and his disdainful greed for money drove him to me again and again. I was often in despair and yet no one could discover my situation. After he had cost me 10,000 francs and another attempt at blackmail had failed, he denounced me to the police. I was arrested immediately, confessed my sexual relationship with my braggart, who is as good an urning as I am! I came to be sentenced to prison. My whole social position was destroyed, my honourable family was brought grief and shame, all friends who had held me in high esteem fell away from me. That was an evil time! And yet I had to say to myself: you have failed, yes, in the face of general morality and in view of what you and your family would have to face if it became known; but I have not failed against nature, a thousand times no, and thus even a part of the other guilt falls from me and on an outmoded law that throws the degenerate voluptuary together with the urning forced to satisfy his urge.

The nature of my sexual satisfaction is not pederasty, but an aid to onanism with simultaneous touching of the sexual part of the other, whereby a healthy, not at all overstimulated, beneficial discharge of semen takes place and I feel well, free and refreshed afterwards.

You can see how natural and original our kind is from the following: About two years ago I was at a friend's house in mixed, merry company. A lively, fun-loving, young, pretty lady, whom I otherwise liked, dressed up in the course of the evening as an officer with a moustache, and from the minute she entered in these metamorphic trousers I felt a sexual attraction. A friend once advised me to marry and dress my wife in men's clothes.

I know of a beautiful relationship between two urnings in Geneva that has existed for more than seven years. Such a relationship is only possible where sensual love is accompanied by respect. If a pledge of such love were also possible, then they would be entitled to marry—but the relevant proposal by Ulrichs is ridiculous.[1]

One thing remains true. Our love, too, produces the most beautiful, noblest blossoms, develops all the nobler instincts and stimulates the spirit, just as in the young man who loves his girl. They find the same devotion, the same willingness to sacrifice, even if they put their lives on hold, the same pain, the same sorrow, the same joy, the same happiness as in the true man. I would also like to add that I am physically fully developed, as far as I can judge, and that there is nothing special to be noticed in my sexual parts. My gait, my voice are both male and one would not normally realise that I am an urning, but many people can tell our species immediately, betrayed by a glance, by the look in our eyes, our gait, posture, the way our body is inclined, the way we sit down on a chair, our clothing and so on.

As a result of my degradation in my homeland, I am now forced to live in America and am not happy with my life here either for fear that people will find out what happened to me in my homeland and therefore despise me. May science succeed in enlightening the people about us unfortunates, but until then there will still be much suffering.

3.2 JP (1885) Bb 1, 37–42

R: *PS4 (1889) Bb 73, PS6 (1891) Bb 96*

My father was the youngest child among 12 siblings, tender and pampered in his youth, nervous and excitable until later in life, in his last years almost constantly tormented by severe headaches, the cause of which was given differently by doctors; my mother died of cerebral typhus in her prime.

Of the relatives on my father's side, I consider a stepbrother of my father (from my grandfather's first marriage), whom I personally no longer knew, to be a decided urning. He was the eldest son and although, if not him, then at least his possible son had an almost certain prospect of owning a beautiful estate, he could not decide to marry, nor to engage in any serious business; he played the aesthete and entertained himself with embroidery. He left the greater part of his fortune to his servant, although a sister, with whom he was on very good terms during his lifetime, was by no means in a favourable financial situation. The words of another of my father's brothers, who once spoke of this same step-uncle in my presence, still ring in my ears: 'Ah, the good brother', he said. 'He was really more woman than man.'

My maternal relatives offer no striking perceptions, at least not to the layman. They are all lively, energetic spirits and I consider them intellectually superior.

I am the third and last child of my parents' marriage, the second died in childhood, my still living elder brother is hypospadias,[2] very weak in character, highly attracted to the opposite sex, talented in poetry and conspicuously absent-minded.

I am 35 years old; I am generally thought to be younger, usually by five or six years of my real age; now my appearance is beginning to keep pace with my age. I am 1.63 metres tall, of weak constitution, but with a blooming complexion; my genitals are quite normal and well formed. My gait and all my movements are quick and lively; I speak quickly, but not fluently, and gesticulate a lot with my hands; I am very embarrassed to speak in public. I am generally shy, very reserved towards strangers and easily embarrassed; I often blush easily and vividly. My great reserve often comes to be interpreted as arrogance, but this is far from me; on the other hand, I am very sensitive to mockery and ridicule.

Sleep and appetite are good; the consumption of coffee and tea in the afternoon or evening excites me and keeps me awake for hours at night; I consume spiritual drinks in very moderate quantities; I avoid tobacco smoking completely, as it does not offer me the slightest pleasure.

Without ever having developed any diligence, I was one of the better pupils at school and have passed all the examinations that a civil servant has to undergo nowadays without any significant effort, without achieving anything extraordinary, for which I lack the necessary calmness and concentration of mind. I believe I possess what the French call *un esprit faux.*[3] I don't see things in a one-sided way, but rather illuminated from all sides. I see the pros and cons; but before the multitude of ideas that come to me when I consider an object, I often lose the ability to distinguish the essential from the unessential. And so, I come to the wrong conclusions.

Sometimes feeling gets the better of reason; in unguarded moments my logic is not the strongest. With others, however, I have a very keen eye for such shortcomings. I have no organisational talent at all, and I would not be useful as a diplomat.

Music, painting, literature, beauty of nature, then traits of kindness of heart and love of humanity find in me a sincere admirer and devotee, while injustice, hypocrisy and presumption, in whatever form they appear, are deeply hateful to me and can outrage me to the utmost; I have a great sense of humour and the comic.

I am a great friend of animals; I divide my excessive tenderness equally between dogs and cats. If I were to keep a dog, I would come to be its slave; but as I am a lover of freedom and any compulsion is unbearable to me, I refrain from acquiring one. It goes without saying that I am an enemy of hunting; I much prefer a stag, a deer, a hare in the wild than in the kitchen.

As far back as I can remember in my childhood, I remember that the lively games of my peers did not attract me very much; when the time came for recreation, I looked for a quiet corner with a book under my arm, where I hungrily devoured fairy tales, stories, travel descriptions, in general everything that fell into my hands that was in print. I was also often to be found in the kitchen. It was a great pleasure for me to be allowed to help the cook; one could especially ingratiate oneself with me through the gift of raw materials in order to cook something oneself with them; the quality of the products of my art was often quite doubtful, since I did not adhere to the tried and tested rules of art, but put my pride in discovering new dishes; even now I like to invent new dishes, at least in my mind.

I spent many an hour sewing, crocheting and embroidering, but I never learned to knit—it bored me. I still embroidered in my university years; I only gave it up when I learned that it was very suspicious and that the expert would immediately smell the urning.

But that's what I am. Since my earliest youth I have felt like a woman. I have never, either waking or dreaming, felt the slightest inclination to touch the most beautiful woman even with the tip of my finger; I have worshipped soldiers for as long as I can remember, formerly without knowing why, now with hot desire. My sexual inclination is through and through that of a woman, my taste roughly that of a Bohemian cook. Handsome soldiers and non-commissioned officers, especially from the cavalry, are incredibly attractive to me sexually; officers and elegant gentlemen not at all. They must be natural boys, sturdy guys with strong muscles, earthy people with simple natures. All who have these qualities find grace before my eyes. A nice, soft, not-too-long moustache increases the attraction of the kiss; I do not like long, full beards. My lovers should not be older than 30, but also not under 20; they must be in full youthful virility to attract me.

From a sexual point of view, women are not only indifferent to me, but also disgusting. To present the female body as the prototype of human beauty is to my mind ridiculous, incomprehensible; I find the bosom disgusting, the female hip formation ugly, unaesthetic. Dancing is therefore an abomination to me; even the smell that the so-called fair sex emits when it is heated by dancing is highly repugnant.

Although I was educated in an institute where I saw and heard many things that could have given me bad ideas, I did not voluntarily ejaculate until I was 26 years old; I instinctively shied away from onanism, although I was very sensually aroused from the beginning of puberty, which, however, came rather late in my case, and the erections often did not want to come to an end; nature helped itself by ejaculating at night under erotic dreams, the subject of which were, of course, only men. In the last years of my stay at the institute, when my comrades went for their daily walks in a row and looked at the passing girls and criticised them, finding them nice and amiable, I could not understand what could be interesting about such a thing, and the conversations about girls bored me to tears. My attention on the walks was captivated by soldiers, grooms, handsome peasant boys and the like. The clatter of spurs attracted my full attention even from a distance, and when the owner approached and was pretty, I almost died of longing. It seemed to me that the highest goal I could aspire to was to fall around the neck of such a lovely creature and kiss it from top to bottom. But even then, as if attracted by a magnet, my eyes were drawn to the genitals, and to be able to touch the forms, which were often clearly visible through tight-fitting breeches, seemed to me to be the greatest delight.

But at that time, I was still quite innocent and naive. I was not aware of the actual sexual nature of this longing; it was only when I went to university and gained full freedom of action that this realisation became clear. Breathlessly, I often pursued a beautiful figure for hours, waiting patiently in front of house doors until they emerged again; when I was sure I had lost sight of them for the day, I hurried home disconsolate, heated and exhausted. With the physical rest then came the mental anguish. I asked myself, why am I not like everyone else? Why did heaven put this terrible passion in my heart? I was boundlessly unhappy and fell asleep with burning tears, only to start the same chase again the next day. I welcomed crowds of people; I often managed to snuggle up to a handsome soldier and press my hand against his genitals; how enraptured I clung to the figure. But despite the momentary happiness, this was still no satisfaction, and my silent lamentation remained inexpressible.

My only consolation was the hope that the urge would come to an end, and that the inclination for girls would come. But of course, it did not come. I often had erections for days on end, I was in the throes of sensual excitement, but it was impossible for me to seek relief in a girl, it went against my nature.

Around the age of 24, I learned from reading Ulrichs's writings that I was not the only man of this kind. I received the writings through a friend who, like me, loves male beings, albeit in a different way. Although he soon made himself known to me, I could not decide to return trust with trust. Apart from great shame, the reason for my reticence was probably also the fact that my tastes are quite different from his. The perverse sexual inclination was now our almost exclusive topic of conversation. I felt a great relief as a result; the earlier inner uneasiness about the bad, immoral nature of my inclination disappeared, and I no longer considered myself worse than any other young person in love; nevertheless, I remained quite unhappy. One evening I was overwhelmed by my agonised state, I could no longer hold on. I had to pour out my heart and revealed myself to another—not the aforementioned—childhood friend. My confidant was quite speechless at my opening. He had never heard or known anything other than that pederasty existed and that it was a shameful vice of worn-out libertines, born of gluttony. My boundless pain at that time must have carried a powerful, convincing force; from that hour on, he believed in the innate love of men for their own sex and has remained my best friend.

Not long afterwards I also revealed myself to my first-mentioned friend. By chance he had made the acquaintance of a young urning who had approached him out of love. We began to study him. He was more feminine than a woman and an interesting object. The poor man later ended up committing suicide in another town; he threw himself into the water. He didn't excite me in the least sexually, but he was the turning point in my sexual life, because he got me my first rendezvous with a soldier.

The first pleasure has since been followed by many others; I have become somewhat calmer, but have a great need for sexual pleasure, which is very beneficial to me physically and mentally. I must constantly have a little love intrigue and the more romantic the love trade, the better. However, circumstances force me to be moderate in everything and I do not exaggerate the pleasure in any way.

In the male body, it is above all the sexual organ that excites me, both the penis and the scrotum, and I make a distinction about the size and beauty of the latter, then strong, round buttocks and firm calves excite me the most. Erection always occurs at the mere sight of my lover, often some time before the tryst; however, semen is only ejaculated after prolonged friction with my sexual organ; merely touching it or even hugging and kissing my lover is not enough for it to occur.

The sexual act regularly consists of mutual masturbation with the hand; but I find the imitation of coitus between the thighs, where I lie on my back and feel completely like a woman and the moment of greatest pleasure comes with ejaculation on the part of my lover.

About two years ago, at the prolonged persuasion of my uranian friend, I went to visit a pretty pleasure girl to test the effect of the naked female body on me. With a silent shudder I lay in bed next to the person. My only thought was, if only I were gone again; I felt not a trace of sensual emotion. Yes, if that had been a man! After a long manipulation on her part, the erection finally occurred and finally also an ejaculation without any pleasure. I jumped from the bed in disgust; instead of the freshness and relief that I feel when dealing with men, I was overcome by a dull fatigue and exhaustion, and I am clearly still conscious of a certain moral dejection, as if I had committed a rather unpleasant act. I have had enough of this one experiment; I am now quite clear about the repulsiveness of the female body.

I cannot find the love of men pathological. I would therefore consider myself perfectly healthy psychologically if I were not haunted and tormented by a strange mania in my sexual life.

The highest, quite irresistible sexual excitement occurs in me when I imagine a handsome, strong man, possibly a soldier, being laid on the bench, and beating him twenty-five times. Cruelty and the deepest pity for the poor fellow fight in my heart, but the result is always the highest sexual excitement. I fight this unfortunate mania as best I can and thank heaven that the time of corporal punishment is over.

By the slightest external inducement, the thought often comes flying; the sight of a bench, of hazelnuts, of an elastic stick, then of things still more distant, is sufficient to come to the inducement of the most violent sensual excitement in consequence of the association of ideas.

The unhappy, certainly morbid passion has also even tempted me to masturbate, since an ejaculation relieves me to a high degree and frees me from these tormenting thoughts. This mania is the only side of my sexual life that embarrasses me; my love for men only gives me many a gloomy hour insofar as I am often seized with a sudden fear that my inclinations might come out in the open, an event that would bring me almost to the brink of despair.

When will people begin to approach the matter without prejudice, even in public? In any case, science must not pause to disseminate the results obtained and make them comprehensible to the layman.

3.3 JP (1885) Bb 2, 42–7

R: *PS4 (1889) Bb 63, PS6 (1891) Bb 89*

Dear Sir,

You wish to have biographies of various urnings. In the interest of science, I have no hesitation in giving you as accurate an autobiography as possible in the following, in which I will endeavour to give all the data that come into consideration here with the greatest possible objectivity.

I am the youngest of 15 siblings (nine from the same mother); two of the siblings died young, the others all grew up normally, except for one brother who got a severe brain inflammation at the age of one-and-a-half years and has remained sickly ever since. This brother is now close to 60 years of age, and I believe he also has an urning disposition. At least, he is the only one of my siblings who has not married and, as far as I know (I have never discussed this subject with him), has never had sexual intercourse with women.

All my other siblings grew up quite normally, all married at an early age and, apart from one sister, are all blessed with more or less large families. (As far as I know, there have never been any mental disorders in the family, neither on my father's nor on my mother's side.)

I, myself, have had a completely normal outward development. I am now 48 years of age. With the exception of gastric complaints, which I suffered from for a while, I have always been healthy. My external appearance is completely male; I am of average height; I am constitutionally and physically strong; early on I had a luxuriant beard, and even my body (chest, arms, legs) is unusually hairy; my gait and movement are decidedly male; my sexual organs are also completely normally developed; my voice is a sonorous, masculine one. In outward appearance, therefore, absolutely nothing of an urning can be detected in me. Mentally, I can say that my development and ability are above the average level. From my earliest youth, I had great ease in learning and, without any effort on my part, I was usually first at school. Later, I also completed my studies with excellent results. From an early age I showed a special talent for the exact sciences, especially for higher mathematics, mechanics and so on, and although I have a completely independent financial background and therefore do not need to earn a living, I always took pleasure in serious studies, which I pursued at university and later with zeal, so that I could be active as a successful scientific writer.

In my environment, I am considered a decidedly clever man, and I do indeed believe that I have a quick and correct view in the assessment of people and circumstances, and that I think logically and correctly. In addition to this decidedly masculine development of the mind, however, certain symptoms of a more feminine nature were also evident in me from my earliest youth. I count among these an unusual softness of disposition, which tends to be very easily moved. At the theatre, it is still highly embarrassing for me when I suddenly burst into tears; I used to be laughed at by my friends because I couldn't watch a drama or read a novel without bursting into tears at the first touching scene.

Another feminine trait in me is a dexterity in my fingers and a delight in female handicrafts that is rare in men. Even as a little boy, I quickly copied the intricate art of knitting, crocheting, embroidery and so on from my sisters, and my greatest joy was when I was able to snatch my mother's or one of my sisters' handiwork unnoticed and continue working on it. Even later—at university and on journeys—if something was defective in my laundry or clothing, I was happy to repair the damage myself. If I didn't think I could use the time I spent on it more usefully, and if I wasn't afraid of making a fool of myself, I would still be happy to do feminine needlework, embroidery and the like. This is probably connected to a pronounced sense and understanding of women's toiletry, so that I am very often consulted in this direction by the ladies of my acquaintance.

As far as the development of my sex drive is concerned, I have always been uranian, as far back as my memory goes. Even as a small boy, handsome men made a much deeper impression on me than beautiful women or girls. The first sexual excitement I remember—although I did not recognise it as such at the time—was towards a tutor who was an extremely handsome man. I was perhaps only nine or 10 years old at the time, and my greatest pleasure was when he allowed me to climb on his knees. I had my first pleasurable sexual sensations without being clear about the details. I remember from that time that when the tutor had gone out, I liked to go to his wardrobe to take in the smell that emanated from his clothes—especially from his trousers. From the same time on, that is, from about my ninth or tenth year, all handsome men attracted my attention, and I especially loved the soldiers. I was particularly captivated by certain outstandingly beautiful officers, and wherever I could, I would try to meet them and follow them unnoticed as often as I could. When I was a boy of perhaps 12 years of age, I had the opportunity, together with other friends, to come into close contact with girls of the same age, so that they showed us their sexual organs; this left me completely cold, while at the same time I already regarded every handsome friend with special interest and followed the soldiers and especially individual handsome officers as often as I could. Even then, I was particularly impressed by very slim figures, and I loved it when they wore their uniforms as close to their bodies as possible—a characteristic that I have retained to this day. At the age of 14, I was in love with a slim, handsome lieutenant. I followed him wherever he went and was happy just to be near him, to hear his voice or even only just to touch his coat with my hand in a crowd, for example, when leaving the theatre, and in a very clever way I often managed to make such touching possible.

At that time, I had no idea that other people could have feelings similar to mine, and naively, I told my tutor that I was in love—but with an officer. I didn't understand his admonition that I shouldn't do that, that it was a grave mistake. As often as I had sexual excitement in my dreams from my earliest childhood onwards, it was always in connection with men, mostly officers, not once with women. As I got older, the more clearly the urning sexual nature developed, without me being able (until much later) to follow my sexual inclinations in any way other than entirely platonically, or rather, with the help of my imagination.

I have already mentioned how much the military and especially handsome officers excited me sexually. Long before I was a man, I immediately got erections when I followed a handsome officer, especially if he wore tight-fitting and taut trousers. It was then enough to exert a little pressure on my genitals with my hand in my trouser pocket to get pleasure—all this before I was a man. I remember very clearly, it was at a big parade, where I was again following a beautiful officer in the usual way and was giving myself the familiar pleasure. I was terribly frightened when I suddenly felt a wetness on my genitals and thought I was bleeding—but it was the first ejaculation I had.

So as I became older and older, I had no idea that there were other people in the world with a very similar disposition. All my peers now turned to intercourse with women. I thought what I was doing was wrong, sinful, and I tried to control myself. I managed, often for months at least, to avoid giving myself sexual pleasure, but in my sleep the same dream images haunted me again and again, and nature procured its rights through pollutions, and this occurred all the more frequently the more I tried to control myself while awake. Finally, I wanted to try to change myself through contact with women—I still thought that the game of my imagination, which always haunted me, was a damnable aberration. Through the mistress of one of my friends, I came to meet a pretty girl—whom everyone was happy to 'deflower'; I was already 21 years of age. We were alone; the girl let all her charms play; we kissed, she pressed me powerfully against her—all in vain. I remained cold, and despite my ardent desire to finally make it equal to all other men, it remained impossible; I had not the slightest erection. A second attempt, which I made a few years later, was exactly the same; only this time I had to deal with a brothel mistress who finally worked my member with her hand until erection came; she finally introduced my member into her cleft and through the mechanical friction I finally brought it to ejaculation. But it was not a real pleasure, and during this coitus I had the sensation as if I had masturbated, while the way in which I had since prepared my own sexual pleasure was decidedly natural according to my disposition and also a far more satisfying pleasure for me.

So, I spent my youthful manhood in a futile struggle against myself and my nature. It was not until I was about 30 years of age that I came across the writings of Numa (Ulrichs), and I cannot describe what a relief it was for me to learn that there were many other men who were just as sexually inclined as I was, and that what I felt sexually was not an aberration but a special sexual disposition inherent in me by nature. For the first time, I experienced the pleasure of finding sexual satisfaction through direct contact with a man's body. I no longer tried in vain to fight against a deeply implanted disposition, and since I have given my urning nature freer rein, I am happier, healthier and more efficient! There is one point that I have not yet touched on and that I would have preferred to skip completely, but to be complete I would like to mention a few things: it concerns my marital life. I have been married for about 15 years. At first, I hoped that regular intercourse with a woman would suppress my urning disposition. I thought that in marriage this would come to be quite different from the first attempts I had made with prostitutes. This hope has not been fulfilled in any way. Even with my spouse, whom I love very much spiritually (not physically), coitus has never been possible for me in a natural way. Erection never occurs as a result of close contact with the female body or as a result of caresses from my wife, but only by imagining as vividly as possible those handsome men who have recently made a lively impression on me, and by imagining them in the positions and clothing that most appeal to me—that is (it is almost always young officers that I imagine in this way), in tight-fitting trousers and tightly laced uniforms, whom I then imagine sitting on my lap or the like. I also achieve the same effect by imagining myself in such clothing, which I then picture in all its details, to then have the officers in question reach out and touch me or the like. As opposed to other urnings, it is a peculiarity of mine that I am less attracted to the naked bodies of men than when I see them in rather close-fitting clothing. Even if I have an erection in this way or by mechanical means, I can only continue the sexual act by continuing to work my imagination in urning images. If I refrain from this for only a moment, even after ejaculation, the erection also disappears; the woman's caresses have no stimulating effect on me whatsoever, but, by hindering my calm immersion in my fantasy images, only disturb me. Under such circumstances it is understandable that coitus, even with a woman I adore and hold in high esteem, has never been a real pleasure for me, but rather a tiresome duty. Fortunately, my wife is not at all sensually inclined; I also prepared her before marriage for the fact that I would have little to offer her in the way of sex (without telling her the internal reason for this). So we have been living in separate bedrooms for some time now, and sexual intercourse in marriage has ceased altogether, to my decided relief.

3.4 PS3 (1888) Bb 33, 81–7

R: *PS4 (1889) Bb 57, PS5 (1890) Bb 68, PS6 (1891) Bb 81*

The only thing I know about my grandparents is that my paternal grandmother died past the age of 80. I have heard nothing about any of them dying of a particularly remarkable illness. My father was an extremely strong, always healthy man, who probably drank many strong spirits, but to my knowledge never got drunk. He had an oft-tried sound mind, was very fierce and was said to have been very sensual in his youth. He died of apoplexy in his seventies. My mother, who gave life to many children, was also a vigorous woman, never ill, of whom I only know that in the last years of her life, she suffered from sometimes aggravated chest pain. She died of liver disease at the age of 79. Of my siblings, two died as small children, one adult sister died when I was quite young of an acute internal disease, one brother died at the age of about 35 of a disease unknown to me, another died of heart disease at the age of about 47. One brother and one sister, who are still alive, sometimes had attacks of nervous excitement as children, my brother probably up to the age of 17, which in individual cases increased to a kind of persecution mania. Now there are no more traces of it. My brother, as well as another older sister, seems to have inherited something of my mother's precordial anxiety, which also afflicts me from time to time.

I am soon to be 50 years old and have never been ill, except for scarlet fever and gastric fever in my childhood. Since then, I have been healthy until, perhaps 10 years ago, a nervous agitation became noticeable. I am absolutely sure that this is only the result of the incidents that are the consequence of my sexual perversity. Moreover, in the vast majority of cases it is not so severe that I could not outwardly master it by exerting my willpower.

I am a tall, strong man with a full beard; the hair on my body is sparse, and I have a mammary formation. I look younger than I am and have a cheerful, as I am told, 'sunny' disposition by nature, which has, of course, been darkened for years when I think of my condition. But I am usually able not to let other people notice this; I also forget my unhappiness when I am in a stimulating, cheerful circle, which I then like to enliven myself, so that I believe I am regarded as a very welcome companion.

No one will come to see that I have a sexual inclination towards men: I dress seriously; my taste in artistic things, with which I occupy myself a great deal, is likewise serious; even though I have not done much physical exercise apart from strenuous and repeated journeys on foot as often as possible in the valleys and mountains, I have no feminine inclinations whatsoever; I have danced much and gladly, only out of pleasure in the rhythmic movement, not out of the desire to come into close contact with a woman; on the contrary, this has always been repugnant to me, especially when I perceived a smell in the process, such as only emanates from a woman.

I always liked to be in the society of women, and it also appealed to me to be sought out there. But it was always only spiritual intercourse that attracted me; I immediately felt violently repelled as soon as anything occurred that could have even remotely aroused sensuality in others. I am considered to be of a humane nature, living at peace with the world and with myself and experiencing the pleasure of inner harmony.

No one around me suspects my inner conflict and my state of complete resignation.

Even I cannot admit, despite being urning, that my nature is a 'morbid' one, or you must also call other whole categories of people who are usually considered normal morbid. No one sees anything morbid in me; I have never heard that there is anything quirky about me nor that I have any peculiarity that might suggest or degenerate into something morbid.

On the contrary, I am considered to be of a calm, deliberative nature; my advice has been sought in many delicate cases, and I have been entrusted with positions of honour which I have not done the least to obtain, and in my profession as a businessman I am considered to be capable. I only lack the inclination to the female sex, just as many people have a pronounced aversion to other things; but since by far the majority of men do not lack this inclination [toward women], and those who actually lack it do not say so, we come to be called 'ill' because we appear to be the invisible minority who suffer from this aversion to sexual intercourse with women, which is completely inexplicable to others.

And we come to be thought ill for another, unfortunately quite valid reason, namely, that we have really become ill, and that cause and effect are then confused. What nerves are required to endure the years of agitation connected with finding a friend with whom one lives in sexual intercourse; to endure the constant fear of discovery and, as a decent human being, to always be aware that one word is enough to be expelled in disgrace forever from the circles in which one socialises comfortably and with respect; what, finally, must we endure when we lack a friend whose sexual intercourse has become absolutely necessary to us to preserve our health, when, with our imagination alone, we finally surrender to onanism. Then, of course, we become ill, as animals are afflicted with rabies if they are prevented from practising the sexual act appropriate to their nature.[4]

When I first made the discovery that I was attracted to my sex in an extraordinary way, I cannot say exactly; in any case, I was not more than six or seven years of age when I induced a playmate of the same age to go with me to a secluded place and show me his sex parts while I did the same, whereupon we played with each other's sex parts. Sometime later I played this game with a relative who was six or seven years older than I, and the end result was soon mutual onanism, which excited me so much that I often created the chance for myself to renew the pleasure.

Soon afterwards, I began an even more enchanting relationship with a second boy, eight years older than I, which, however, did not last long, while the former, often interrupted by long periods of time, lasted until my twenty-second year. However, since I met him once a week in the best case, and often much less frequently, I became addicted to onanism, which I did very frequently for years and unfortunately still do today, although somewhat less frequently and only when I have no young man to satisfy me. How I stand in relation to my affection for the male sex was only to come to me completely when I was about 18 years of age and met a cousin of mine, a beautiful boy of about 13–14 years. At the sight of him I was overcome by such a blissful feeling, I began to tremble violently all over my body, while the blood rose to my head, that those around me thought I had become unwell.

I sought every opportunity to meet him, but an insurmountable shyness prevented me from approaching him or even disclosing myself to him. He must have recognised my infatuation for him, for he soon approached me in a confidential manner, at which moment my excitement was renewed in the same way. Soon after, we left each other without the relationship being anything other than platonic. But from him my innermost being had become clear to me.

When I was 20 years of age, I came to live with a young man of 18 in a boarding house. We liked each other, and after only a few days I came to be his bedfellow; for the first time I had the happiness of being able to hold a beloved young man in my arms and feel at one with him in blissful love. We always satisfied each other by imitating coitus between our thighs, almost every night. Unfortunately, the relationship only lasted through one winter and two summers, then I moved away and lost this friend forever. In the meantime, a few books by Numa Numantius[5] had fallen into my hands, and from these I received the explanation of my condition, which until then was still completely inexplicable to me. I wanted to put an end to this by visiting the rooms of prostitutes with other young people. I shivered at the thought, but I drank a little courage into myself, and the presence of the friends prevented me from turning back at the door, which I would undoubtedly have done if I had been alone. So it happened three times that I forced myself on a woman, and just as often I had to leave without having done anything, because an erection could not be achieved at all. The first time I took a girl to my flat in the hope that I, safe from disturbance and not bound to a certain time, would bring her to coitus sooner. The result, in spite of the girl's kind complaisance, was exactly the same negative. When I was a soldier, I lived on the same floor of a girl who was kept by a merchant. She asked me to visit her at a time when we would be quite safe. I did so, determined to use all my imagination to finally reach my goal. The success was pitiful. The very moment I embraced her to proceed to coitus, I was seized with a chill, a tremor in all my limbs, a horror that, still willing to conquer it, I finally came to feel really pale and unwell and had to withdraw. A few years later (I might have been 27), I once again wanted to give myself a chance to change my mind about sex. I had heard that a girl was madly in love with me and desperately wanted to give herself to me.

We had a rendezvous in my flat, hoping that I would have different feelings towards a girl who came to me out of love. After the first fiery lovemaking sessions, it almost seemed as if I was going to warm up, but from the moment I began to think of the coitus that was to follow, everything came to an end, the same rigid frost as in earlier cases set in: my role was played out. With moral aphorisms I dismissed those who were aroused to the core. Since that time, I have given up such attempts. In all cases, the specific smell of women has contributed to increasing my horror. When I see a pretty young man between 15 and 18 years of age, it can happen that I forget the time and place, that I do everything in my power to get a glimpse of him or to speak to him, often under the most stupid pretexts. My being goes into a feverish excitement, and I am completely indifferent to anything else in the world but holding on to the moment. Girls, at the sight of whom my friends become dithyrambic, leave me cold; just having to think about them bores me in short order. In my twenty-fifth year, I came to a distant town and saw a young man of 18 there whose sight inflamed me and whom I had to get to know at all costs. After some difficulties, I managed to persuade him to visit me. I was seriously feverish when he entered. He had noticed my extraordinary affection; I approached him tenderly, and he softened; I just thought I had my beloved when a door slammed next door. He started up, came to, and the opportunity was over. He had retired to a family where, by chance, there was still a vacancy; I moved there and lived for nine months separated only by an open door from the object of my longing; at noon we ate alone together. The first days we spent together in this way were days of the purest bliss for me, when I asked for nothing more from life. I felt the urge to possess my beloved, but this was never to come to pass: when I came home late at night, he was half undressed or only in his underclothes on my sofa or even asleep on my bed. Awakened, he tolerated my lying down next to him and caressing him; if I wanted more, he jumped up and rushed to his room. And this game was repeated for months. The torment I endured finally seemed unbearable to me; the fantasies that took shape in my brain were terrible, they could turn me into a criminal against my lover, they could also lead me to madness. But I survived this time, admittedly with a loss in my health and my mood. At that time, I may have laid the foundation for my nervous upsets, for the head pressure that plagued me for a long time and for the resignation that is the basic feature of my mood today. That was one of those experiences that can make an urning 'morbid'. I changed my place of residence and moved to a larger city in Belgium, where I live. The son of a couple who were close friends of mine, a boy of about 14 years, quickly joined me and soon came to be my lover. A relationship developed out of this, which, from my point of view, I must call 'as ideal' as any may ever have been at the time of the flowering of ancient Hellas; indeed, I would go further and say that the boy's father, if he had known our true relationship, would perhaps have had to think very hard about destroying it, if he had paid attention to how the boy developed as a result of my friendship. He was flabby, lazy, not considered very talented, but his good character and his kindness secured him the friendship of those around him, so that he came to be treated half affectionately, half like a Cinderella. Very soon he opened his whole heart to me. He confessed to me that he had been masturbating daily for some time; I drew his attention to the consequences that his passion could, indeed must, finally have and asked him to be content with sexual intercourse with me. I would like to add that for the whole time of its duration of about seven years, it consisted exclusively of imitating coitus between the thighs.

He followed my advice, and at first had returned only sometimes to onanism. I tried to interest him in many things and was pleased to see how he made an effort to learn about the things that interested me the most at various times. It gradually helped that I aroused in him the ambition to achieve a place among the better ones at school. He got on easily at school, his whole nature had become determined and he also tried to acquire my ease of movement in ladies' circles, even if I had to prod him hard at first. Today he is a respected businessman, married, without contrary sexual feelings; our friendship, however, continues in unchanged cordiality, even if our former relationship has long since ceased.

I was not granted the opportunity to enter into a similar relationship a second time. It is true that another, rarely intelligent, boy of precocious energy joined me in the same way. He, too, opened his whole heart to me and felt highly honoured by my friendship, which he showed me by the greatest attachment, but I only got him to give himself to me once, then never again, so that I finally gave up the attempts, but remained attached to him in friendship. A strong, well-developed boy, aged 15, also approached me; indeed, it was he who forced himself on me. He visited me twice without being asked. Since I was known in his family but felt that I had little in common with them, I did not want to enter into an intimate relationship with him, even though he appealed to me physically. He sat down next to me on a couch, lay over me, embraced my neck and rested his head against my cheek. When I, barely able to contain my excitement, touched his thighs, he opened them, and when I then grasped his genitals, he sank over me as if fainting.

But I didn't want to deceive him, because I felt inside that I couldn't be his devoted friend, so I raised him up and told him that he should realise where this would lead. He left, but after a few days, at a time when he knew I was coming home, he met me on the street in front of my flat and followed me in. He started the same game again, which finally paralysed my willpower and ended with us lying in my bed undressed. Now he knew how to get me to perform anal sex by making movements, and at the same time masturbating him. This was disgusting to me, but with his voluptuous actions I finally had the same pleasure. I asked him if he had already had intercourse with men in this way, but he firmly denied it, so that I must assume that he had heard something about it at school.

Our intercourse, which remained purely sexual without closer friendship, lasted from two to eight years and alternated in form with the way he wanted and the way I had hitherto practised, but the latter remained predominant by far, because I do not like the former and have not practised it again.

From now on, unfortunately, I can only report on relationships that I have established with young people who are intellectually beneath me. Only once, a year-and-a-half ago, did a young person who was related to me and whom I liked in every respect approach me in such a way that it would have been easy for me to make him inclined towards my intentions. But reasons partly of his person and partly of my family kept me from doing so, even though it came to me with great difficulty. Among all the people with whom I have been in contact for the last 14 years—there have been five of them—there is one urning. As I lay in bed, while he was sitting on the bed, touching his thighs and his genitals, I noticed by his trembling excitement and by the seething, will-less devotion that here I had before me a different nature from that of my former lovers. He lay down with me, his whole body trembling as he embraced me fervently. The relationship between us continues in the same way today after 11 years—he is now 27 years of age. We love each other dearly; I have influenced his course of education and have also achieved relatively good results. He is outwardly a good-looking person, of decent character and really devoted to me. But since we can't get together as often as his nature demands, he has had to enter into a few other relationships with young subordinate people, which are always soon resolved. He has always told me this. He feels just as repelled by women as I do, even though he has performed coitus with women a few times. So now I stand lonely in the world, not understanding why I don't marry, since I have all the qualities to be a happy family man. I am envied because of some of my abilities, which pave the way for me in social life; I have a large circle of acquaintances and friends who show me goodwill in a city where I am known to the majority by name and person and where I am respected, outwardly happy and seemingly satisfied with my fate, and inwardly so desolate that I have long since renounced all the pleasures of life. I envy the worker who goes for a walk on Sundays with his wife and child and is allowed to show the world his small and, for him, often his greatest, only happiness, who, if he is otherwise a decent person, does not need to hide anything in the depths of his soul and who, when he suffers, may openly be confident in the humanity of people.

When I see how the well-situated citizen has a firm foundation in his home, in his family, in which he anchors his heart, on which he builds a happiness in life that fills his soul, a happiness that he exerts all his strength to increase and in which he basks before the world with a satisfied expression, and I see myself standing beside him as an outcast pariah and my world sinking into ruins, then come moments when I am seized by despair, when I ask why nature has formed me in this way, with powers and abilities, including those for thinking about my destiny, and alongside this with this inability to build a life for myself on foundations in keeping with nature. But not enough that I must do without this happiness, no, I must also be hunted like a deer, must always fear that some rascal will denounce me or suspect me in society, and suffer torment if I cannot satisfy my elementary urge. I am also forced to lead a life of lies, I have to pretend to be happy and seem to feel quite like others in conversations about sexual matters. And yet lying is one of the very ugliest things to me. Truly, I would have long since put an end to my sad life if religion, the last supreme comforter, did not prevent me from doing so. But now I will come to terms with life. For the aims that others strive for, to make a name for themselves, to gain an outstanding position externally, to promote a widespread enterprise, for these aims, which ambition helps to come close to, I have become dull; yet I do not know whether in the midst of my striving I will not be recognised as a criminal away from whom society flees far, and who would therefore do better to flee it. If I were to face the law differently, then perhaps I would be able to regain the courage to live, even if I must do without the happiness of seeing dear children grow up. Dear Professor! You will be able to feel with me what it means to have to close in on myself all my life what touches me most deeply in life and to be able to confide in no one, while I have so often been the confidant in the greatest joy and deepest sorrow. You are the first to whom I open myself. Make use of this letter in any way you wish. Perhaps it will one day contribute to making the fate of those born later, to whom nature has given the same feelings as me, easier.

3.5 PS5 (1890) Bb 76, 155–61

R: *PS6 (1891) Bb 87*

My mother, with the exception of a temporary headache that lasts no more than a day, is perfectly healthy and full of indestructible *joie de vivre*, cheerfulness and is creative when it comes to painting and music. As far as I know, both of my grandparents were mentally normal.

I am the first-born of the family. My brother, a year younger, suffers from sexual anaesthesia even now. As he tells me, he has had pollutions only twice but without voluptuous sensation. Masturbation, although he knows its nature, leaves him cold, just as little is he interested in girls in his sleepy indifference. Of my sisters, the older one (15 years of age) seems to me to be of the same type in this respect, whereas the younger one (12 years of age) shows an early and extremely lively sexual feeling. As I noticed, my mother found out a long time ago that she masturbates, probably as a result of seduction.

I already showed sexual receptivity in my third year. I remember such episodes with particular accuracy. For example, I often tried to look up women's skirts, loved to follow our coachman's son to the privy and stroke his naked anus and once tried to touch the genitals of a 12-year-old boy friend of mine at the urinal. In my fifth year, a lively inclination for a playmate of the same age awoke for the first time. My most ardent wish was to embrace and kiss him, but I did not dare to do so for fear of being laughed at.

In an institute where I received my first school lessons and, as I may well say, showed myself to be a quite well-disposed pupil, I soon began to love several classmates passionately one after the other. One boy, with whom I had a great deal of contact, but only on a purely companionship basis, showed feelings of the same vivacity towards his friends, and we almost systematically joined together to make each other's lovers inclined by praising the lover and hinting at his inclination, which, by the way, we only rarely succeeded in doing. Only once did I succeed in having a lover give me a kiss in all naivety after long preparations, the highest thing I hoped to achieve. In my dreams, even then, I used to press my beloved friends against me filled with ardent love. The sexual moment had completely receded into the background during those years.

When I was nine, I went to a boarding school during my parents' stay in the south. Here, too, I soon fell in love with one fellow, soon with another. Delicate, slender boys with finely cut faces, lively natures and, above all, nice clothes were the only ones who aroused my interest. But for a long time, because of my timidity, I could only achieve friendships like everyone else, never kisses and embraces. If I could put my arm around my friend's neck, then I was already happy. Masturbation, solitary and mutual, was, as I later learned, very common in the dormitories; I had not yet been let in on the pleasurable secret because of my shy seclusion. Nevertheless, I was eager to feel the genitals of my comrades and tried to catch a glimpse of them wherever I could. I sometimes heard people telling each other with mysterious indignation that one or the other had been caught playing with his 'thing', but I couldn't enjoy it because I didn't know the friction. As time went by and I grew up, I became a little bolder in my courtship, so that at the age of 14 I enjoyed the unspeakable happiness of embracing and kissing a lover with whom I found reciprocal love. Soon, however, I became tired of him and turned my affections to others again. I left the boarding school with my confirmation, not without joy, since I had had to endure much ridicule because of my soft and timid nature. I only want to remember one fact. During a stay at the seaside resort, I experienced the much-vaunted 'time of first love', that is, that of the opposite sex. It occurred one after the other with three little girls I had met at the children's ball, but it was much weaker and of shorter duration than my passion for my friends. I also wondered how this love could be praised so much more highly than friendship.

After my confirmation, I entered the upper third of a grammar school and at the same time was enrolled in a teacher's boarding house. I was very active intellectually, occupied myself a lot with artistic and religious questions and later even decided to convert to Catholicism. But all too soon, complete unbelief replaced my pietistic enthusiasm and led me into the arms of Hartmann's and Darwin's teachings, which I still study with lively interest and calm scientific seriousness. At that time, I was seduced for the first time by one of my fellow boarders into onanism, from which I have not yet been able to tear myself away, despite my temporary efforts to do so. I entered into lively sexual intercourse with my two room-mates, who were partly willing to engage in mutual masturbation and partly reluctant to do so, like my brother, whom I also did not spare as the fourth and whom I even now occasionally abuse. For [*LATIN: ejaculation*], only the sensation of lust heightened by touching the other's penis was sufficient. Pollution soon set in, perhaps because my genitals were already as mature as a man's. My hair was also already well advanced, especially on my upper and lower legs, anus and pubic area. Now my armpits, the skin along my abdomen, my upper lip and chin, but not my chest, are also very hairy. I did not find a lover at that time, because most of the visitors to the grammar school belonged to the lower classes and did not suit my pampered tastes. Besides, a handsome comrade from my old boarding school, whom I had only been allowed to love platonically, still lived in my memory, and I made him the hero of a 'student novella'. In it, I tried to portray the love life at the institute, which I did not indulge in alone.

After a two-year stay, I left this grammar school for another one in the city where my mother had married for the second time; that is, where my stepfather lived. Although I always looked pale because of my lung weakness (I had only really been ill with scarlet fever and measles), my appearance must have really changed; in short, I noticed from my parents' insinuations that they thought I was a masturbator and now anxiously tried to avoid this appearance. In response to a direct question from my mother, I presented myself quite innocently. Again, I began to glow for several pupils, but because they were all far from me to no avail. I even noticed that it was now mainly younger boys who interested me, that I always felt I was in an active courting role, but that I was free of sexual needs towards them. I quickly came to terms with a slight lung catarrh, but on examination by the doctor I was sent into healthier air. So I entered the prima of a grammar school as an alumnus, and here I was to spend the best part of my life.

Fornication and these landscapes of unnatural debauchery, even between sexually healthy people, being no longer regarded as something illicit among the alumni finally offered me again what I had painfully missed for a whole year. Except it remained confined to mutual onanism and intercrural sex; anal intercourse, which I now learned about for the first time with disgust and revulsion, was known but not practised. The younger pupils, who were placed under the supervision of the older ones, secretly fornicated together in their beds before the 'seniors' went to sleep. If they got caught, they were given moral sermons and probably also a beating. But the older ones, many of whom were quite heterosexual and regularly performed coitus, did not do any better themselves, but visited each other in bed, sometimes dressed, sometimes only in their shirts. I, too, often had such visits and, even if an unloved person lay over me to imitate coitus, I was able to embrace and kiss them for the duration of the act in surging sensual love. After I had tried for about a year without success to get some 12–16-year-old boys (even today I don't go beyond that age)—I had sat for hours chatting with them, even had held them on my lap, but had never dared to kiss them—I finally found a handsome boy in F., who had also loved boys. I made love to him and now began the most beautiful time of my life. Soon we were sitting or lying on the long 'lounge chairs' that replaced the sofas in our bare alumnus rooms, kissing and cuddling each other, and soon we were indulging in experiences and speculations about our strange condition. Only in Hellenic antiquity did we find like-minded people among the philosophers and poets. We knew old love songs, such as Theognis's *Knaben zu lieben ist Wonne* (To love boys is bliss), by heart from reading them often. This love affair was the first time I got to know jealousy. A third urning, named W. (from a highly stressed family), also loved my chosen one and tried to get between us, which he sometimes succeeded in doing, since my views did not harmonise at all with F.'s and I was often angry with him. Nevertheless, I managed to seduce him as often as I wanted. Just as he gave himself to me, he also gave himself to everyone else who wanted to possess him, so that later he was just called 'the whore'. Despite all my passion, I have never been able to respect him, for it is a peculiarity of my condition that beloved boys whom I also respect because of their honour and moral purity never excite me sexually in the slightest way.

After I had completely broken up with F., I fell in love with two charming boys at the same time. I did not love one more than the other, and yet I was lucky enough to come to be loved by both of them in return. My relationship with them always remained a pure one. I helped the fourths with my knowledge where they lacked it, read the German classics with them in the evening or talked to them as if playing a game about everything they needed to know or that could be useful to them. During the day, I had them in my parlour and couldn't kiss and hug them enough. They also returned my caresses from time to time, partly because they really did love me a little, as I believe, and partly because I fulfilled all their wishes, which I could see in their eyes. In the evening I visited them at their bedsides to begin the caresses anew and to leave them only late at night. I might not have been able to stand the teasing of my comrades if I had not, in the course of time, become accustomed to the tone and manner of a light-hearted libertine, so that the whole activity resembled a boisterous sport. In addition, there were four or five other lovers among the 120 pupils, whose relationship was more or less known. The teachers didn't seem to notice or want to notice any of this; at least, they never made a remark. However, one of my last two lovers told me that even a teacher, who seemed to me to be an urning, despite his reluctance, had kissed him passionately. It was the same with me and some of my fellow pupils at the boarding school mentioned above. I still remember how astonished we were that the teacher often caressed the most naughty and lazy pupils so warmly. And it was precisely these lovers who, under the mask of the teacher, used to find out about their 'friendships' and 'sins against the sixth commandment'. When, at Easter 1888, I was to reach the long-awaited goal of the matura examination without having done any work for all the joys of my happy love, I would have preferred to fail in order to extend for half a year longer the happiness that I was now to leave. But I passed, even with distinction, celebrated a happy and sad farewell party with champagne and sweets, and left the house I had grown to love.

But the much-vaunted Freshers Week and the first semester were now for me only a series of endlessly dull days and restless nights during which I dreamed of my abandoned loved ones, whom I was never to see again. I had no interest in girls; I did not know how to find boys for my purposes. I did not yet know the name of my illness; I only knew that I was different from all the others of my sex. In general, I considered myself a pederast. Often, in my ardent need for love, I burst into tears of despair, then I searched for hours in scientific and scholarly books for explanations or analogous phenomena. But only here and there did I notice something of the sort. For example, an acquaintance told me that a man lived one floor above him who always gathered little boys around him, caressed them and exhibited in front of them while singing lewd songs. Another time, I heard from a pupil that in M., one of the most famous alumni, a fraternity had been discovered that enjoyed [*GREEK: children*] after the example of the ancient Hellenes. A teacher had found them: the older ones had lain together with their younger boys, carousing and kissing.

I heard such and similar stories from time to time, but the name 'urning' and the basic nature of urning love were still completely unknown to me. As I sat studying alone in the small, cheerful university town without any acquaintances or friends, I was so passionately overcome by longing for my loved ones that I decided to go and visit them. Once again, 14 days of the old happy love time returned; then I said goodbye for the second time and had to content myself until now with receiving news about my beloved boys from time to time from W., my old rival, who has come to me as something like a friend through the commonality of our feelings and experiences. But I hear that they are already beginning to forget me and no longer want to know anything about me.

So now I am living the most beautiful part of my life, my student days, in desolation. I feel no joy as happiness, no pleasure as enjoyment, since I lack the highest joy, the highest enjoyment, the love that young people need most to thrive. I have found a few acquaintances here, in my second university town; but since I find no pleasure in carousing and their constant conversations about decent or indecent, pretty or ugly girls arouse boredom, if not envy, there is a gulf between us that we feel vividly without speaking of it. They very well have the unconscious feeling that I do not belong in their circle. When I go for a walk alone, I stand in front of the grammar schools or look at the passing boys in the evening, always in the hopeless hope of finding one by chance whom I could take into my room, embrace and kiss like my old lovers.

So far, however, I have not discovered anyone. Following the advice in *Psychopathia Sexualis*, I have tried to wean myself off the love for boys and substitute girls. But the girls of good society are so boring to me with their conventional reserve or their stereotypical coquetry, those of bad society so repulsive in their body fat and soul dirt that my willpower has already flagged. I once attempted coitus in a brothel. After futile friction on the part of the [*LATIN: girl*], my hand finally reached the erection, whereupon the [*LATIN: penetration with the penis*] succeeded without obstacles, but with only slight pleasure. But I lost the desire for the act.

I would like to give a few more indications, as far as I am able to judge them, about my mental and emotional state. I work with pleasure and success in my studies; only when I have brooded and lamented over my abnormal (hence unnatural, morbid) condition, which I still do often enough, does my already weak willpower flag for some time and I only find satisfaction in dreaming about my past happiness and in reading urning novels and autobiographies in *Psychopathia Sexualis.* My interest in artistic matters has waned and given way to more practical studies. I have become much more sober with time, especially in the last few months, and have acquired, as they say, quite a skill in conversation. The latter likes to play into the satirical or frivolous, and in casual company often into the cynical. Pessimistic world-weariness, mocking self-irony and yet a truly honest enthusiasm for justice and morality, although deeds often fail to follow the weak will, sometimes remind me of Heine, whose nature I possess in many ways, but not genius.[6]

Physically I am very well; I feel no unpleasant consequences of the onanism I indulge in twice a week on average, nor of neurasthenic complaints; of physical exercises I do gymnastics, dancing, swimming and fencing, but because of my lack of strength and dexterity I do not particularly enjoy them. My figure is slender, of medium height, very hairy. Apart from an excellent pelvis, I cannot notice any abnormal development of individual parts of my body. So I see in myself a person who feels sexually abnormal and certainly pathological, but only in a sexual sense. I maintain with the majority of all urnings that our sexual abnormality is of no or only secondary importance for our mental state and that we should not be deprived, by law, of the boys and men who are willing to help us in our natural need, which, although abnormal, is certainly no less vital, any more than the lame man should be deprived of his crutch.

3.6 PS5 (1890) Bb 77, 161–4

R: *PS6 (1891) Bb 88, PS7 (1892) Bb 114, PS8 (1893) Bb 114*

Although I have never met other urnings, I am fully informed about my condition, as I have managed to obtain almost all the relevant literature over the years. Recently I also came across your work *Psychopathia Sexualis.*

I saw from it that you consider and research without prejudice, in the interest of science and humanity.

Even if I cannot tell you much of what is new, I will nevertheless talk about some things that you will kindly accept as a further building block of your work, and which I trustingly place in your hands, together with our social salvation.

If you assume that there is often a hereditary strain among us, that may be the right thing to do. My father suffered from a spinal-cord disease even before I was born, later became mentally ill and took his own life.

Another question, which I rather doubt, however, is the view expressed by you in another place that masturbation performed at a young age could lead to a perverted urge.

I, myself (merchant, owner of a small shop), of course unmarried, am currently in my early thirties, outwardly apparently healthy, hardly deviating from the normal male type. I felt my first sexual impulses, equally and exclusively directed towards the male sex, from about the age of 10. From the age of 12 I masturbated. Since coitus with a woman was always absolutely impossible for me despite all attempts, since there was never any desire towards any woman, but rather disgust, and thus never even the slightest erection, I had to satisfy myself exclusively by masturbation up to this day.

If I am to make a confession about the nature of my sexual gratification, I must say that in the past I was sexually stimulated by schoolmates, peers and so on. Now my urge remains towards boys of at least 10, but mostly towards young boys of 15–20.

Above all, I have been attracted for a long time by the strong, healthy and yet fine body shapes of the cadets, whose tasteful uniforms and fine natures particularly excite me. I have no opportunity to come into close, even the remotest, purely social contact with them. It must be enough for me to follow them in the streets and squares, or, in a more favourable case, be it in a pub, on a horse-drawn tram or railway and so on, I may sit close to them and, if I can do so unnoticed, satisfy myself onanistically. My hottest wish would often be to approach such a young man as a friend, servant or slave. Direct pederasty is never on my mind; what I would like is physical touch, embrace, touching of my member on the part of the beloved young man, a kiss on his sexual parts or his buttocks on my part.

But I often have the kind of desire that Sacher-Masoch describes in his *Venus in Pelz* [Venus in Furs]. There, a man voluntarily makes himself the slave of a woman and feels deep shivers of lust when he comes to be chastised and humiliated by her. Only, of course, I feel that I do not want to be the slave of a woman, but only of a man, or rather of a young man, whom I love so infinitely that I would like to surrender to him with my whole being, whether in mercy or in disgrace. These are the images of desire that come to my mind when I visualise the young man or men I have just seen.

I always feel that this onanism is a sad and imperfect stopgap.

In a dream of lust, I proceed in such a way (and I say everything here because I only want to write what is entirely true) that I believe myself to be bound to total obedience to such a young man who pleases me physically. I imagine that he wants to humiliate me and demands of me, for example, that I kiss his feet or smell his sweaty stockings. In the absence of the desired reality, I take my own stockings, smell them, take them into my mouth and then slip them over my genitals, where erection soon follows and ejaculation occurs with a shudder of lust.

Yes, I have even gone so far in these images that I imagined that the young man I had in mind, thought of as my master, would order me to eat his faeces as a humiliation. Again, in the absence of the thought, I then eat of my own faeces, admittedly only in small quantities. With partial disgust and violent palpitations, a strong erection and ejaculation take place.

However, I usually only get to this dirty level of feverish images and their execution if I have not been able to satisfy myself masturbating in the immediate vicinity of a young man for a very long time. This is the more natural thing for me, because then I have a little more pleasure and also some real physical and mental refreshment, even if my ideal of real direct satisfaction in mutual consent has never come to me.

I almost believe that the above horrible fantasies are only the consequence of the normal satiation that is always lacking, that is, of the satisfaction that is normal for me as an urning, that with a regular satisfaction of body against body, the fantasy that is so pricked to the point of madness would calm down and, in any case, would renounce such extravagances. Or equally: it is the final effect of attempted abstinence, for only after a longer period of this kind do these great voluptuous images occur.

I even believe that I would be capable of great, even noble love and sacrifice under different social circumstances. My thoughts are by no means exclusively physical or morbidly sensual. How often a deep rapturous mood seizes me at the sight of a handsome young man, and I pray, as it were, Heine's wonderful words: *You are like a flower, so lovely, so beautiful, so pure* and so on.

And when I once had to part with a young man who respected and appreciated me as his friendly patron, even if my love always remained unknown to him, I could not get the wonderful Scheffel[7] verses out of my mind, the last of which—mutatis mutandis—particularly resounded in my soul:

Grey as the sky the world stands before me.
But turn it for good or evil,
You, dear friend, in faithfulness I think of you!
God bless you! It would have been too beautiful.
God bless you, it was not meant to be!

No young man has ever suspected my love for him, I have never approached anyone in a corrupt or morally harmful way, but I have paved the way for many a one here and there; I spare no effort then and make sacrifices as I can only make them.

When I have the opportunity to have a beloved friend around me, to educate him, to hold him and to support him, when my unrecognised love finds a (naturally sexless) counter-love, then all dirty fantasy images depart from me more and more. Then my love comes to be almost platonic and ennobles itself, only to sink back into the mud when it has been deprived of its dignified betrothal.

Incidentally, I am not one of the worst people, and I can say this without exaggerating myself. More intellectually active than most average people, I take part in everything that moves humanity. I am good-natured, soft and easily moved to pity, cannot harm any animal, let alone a human being; on the contrary, I work well and humanely wherever and however I can.

Even if I cannot reproach myself in the eyes of my own moral conscience and must resolutely reject the world's judgement of us, I still suffer greatly. Although I have done no harm to anyone and consider my love in its nobler practice to be just as sacred as that of normal people, I often suffer severely to the point of weariness of life from the unfortunate fate that intolerance and ignorance bestow upon us.

To describe all the misery, to describe all the unhappy situations, the constant fear of being recognised as odd and facing exclusion from society, all this is probably not possible for any pen or eloquence. The thought of losing one's existence as soon as one is discovered and of being cast out by everyone is more agonising than one might think. Then everything,

everything that one has ever done good would be forgotten; in the feeling of one's great morality every normally inclined person would puff himself up, even if he himself had acted so frivolously in regard to his love. I know many a person of normal disposition whose frivolity in the opinion of his love remains difficult for me to understand.

But what is our misery! We can end our unhappy lives with a curse on humanity. Truly I often long for the peace of the madhouse, and my life may end when it will, the sooner the better; I am ready.

Moving on to another point, I too, like the others who wrote to you, believe that our nervousness is essentially caused only by our unhappy, unspeakably miserable lives within society.

And now one more thing: at the end of your work, you write about the repeal of the legal paragraphs in question. Humanity would certainly not come to ruin even if they were fully repealed. As far as I know, there is no such paragraph in Italy. And in the end, Italy is not a wilderness, but a cultivated country.

I, myself, who must undermine my health in masturbation, could not yet be affected by the law, for example, since up to now I have not violated its letter. But I still suffer from the curse-worthy contempt that weighs upon us. But how is society's view to change as long as a paragraph of law reinforces its immorality? The law should, of course, correspond to the will of the people, but not to the erroneous popular sentiment, and certainly only to that view which the best thinking and scientifically qualified circles of the people cherish, and not to the wishes and preconceived opinions of a sinister mob delusion. And truly insightful minds can no longer persist in the old view in this respect.

Excuse me, Professor, if I close without being named. Do not inquire after me. I could not report anything further of importance. I am handing these lines over to you in the interest of future fellow sufferers. In the interest of science, truth and justice, publish whatever seems appropriate to you.

3.7 PS5 (1890) Bb 80, 170–5

R: *PS6 (1891) Bb 90, PS7 (1892) Bb 115, PS8 (1893) Bb 115, PS9 (1894) Bb 111, PS11 (1901) Bb 143*

When I entered a public school at the age of seven, I felt extremely uncomfortable and found very little acceptance from my fellow pupils. Only one of them, who was a very pretty child, attracted me, and I loved him almost passionately. In the children's games I always knew how to arrange to appear in girls' clothing, and the greatest pleasure for me was to give our maids quite complicated haircuts. I often regretted not being a girl.

My sex drive awoke when I was 13 years of age, and from the moment it arose it was directed towards young, strong men. At first, I was not really aware that this was an abnormality, but the awareness came when I saw and heard what my peers were like in sexual terms. I started masturbating at the age of 13. At the age of 17, I left my parents' home and attended the grammar school of a larger capital city, where I came to live as a boarding pupil with a married grammar schoolteacher, with whose son I subsequently had sexual intercourse. This was the first time I felt sexual satisfaction. I subsequently met a young artist there who very soon noticed that I was abnormal and who confessed to me that the same was the case with him. I learned from him that this abnormality was very common, and this information invalidated my often deeply saddened opinion that I alone was abnormal. This young man had an extensive circle of similar acquaintances, into which he introduced me. There I came to be the object of everyone's attention, since physically, as everyone claimed, I was very promising. I soon came to be idolised and loved by an older gentleman, but I did not find him to my taste and only listened to him for a short time, only to give ear to a younger, very handsome officer who lay at my feet. This was my first love.

After I had passed the matura examination at the age of 19, freed from the constraints of school, I got to know a large number of people who were like or similar to me, including Karl Ulrichs (Numa Numantius).

When I later went on to study medicine and socialised with many normal young people, I was often in the position of having to comply with the request to go to public prostitutes. After I had thoroughly disgraced myself with various women, some of them very beautiful, the opinion spread among my acquaintances that I was impotent, and I fed this gossip by telling them about my alleged exaggerated performances with women. I had a lot of foreign relations at that time, who praised my physique in their circles to such an extent that I was considered an outstanding beauty in wider circles. As a result, someone would arrive at any moment, and I would receive so many love letters that I was often embarrassed. This phenomenon reached its climax when I later lived in the hospital as a doctor for a year. Things went on and off there, like a celebrated personality, and the jealous scenes that took place there for my sake almost led to the discovery of the whole story. Shortly afterwards I fell ill with an inflammation of the shoulder joint, from which I only recovered after three months. In the course of this I had received subcutaneous injections of morphine several times a day, which suddenly came to an end and which I continued in secret after my recovery. For the purpose of special studies, I stayed for some months in Vienna before entering independent practice, where I had access to various circles of my peers through some recommendations. There I made the observation that the abnormality in question, in its very different forms, is just as widespread in the lower classes of people as in the higher ones, and that those who are accessible commercially, for a fee, are also not seldom encountered in the higher classes.

When I settled in the country as a doctor, I hoped to be able to get rid of morphine by means of cocaine, and so I fell into cocaine addiction, which could only be permanently eliminated after three relapses (21 months ago). In my position it was impossible for me to find sexual satisfaction, and I was therefore pleased to see that the use of cocaine resulted in the extinction of my desires. When I was first freed from cocaine addiction under the energetic care of my mother, I went away for a few weeks to recover. The perverse desires had reawakened in all their strength, and when one evening I had amused myself with a man in the open air outside the city, the next day the public prosecutor told me that I had been observed and that charges had been brought against me, but that the act with which I was charged was not punishable according to a decision of the highest court in the German Empire.[8] However, I should be careful, as the news of the incident had already reached the widest circles. I felt compelled to leave Germany after this event and to seek a new home where neither the law nor public opinion would oppose what, like all abnormal impulses, cannot be suppressed by willpower. As I was not for a moment unaware that my inclinations were in opposition to social views, I repeatedly tried to master them, but I only increased them through this, and the same observation was communicated to me by acquaintances. Since I was attracted exclusively to strong, youthful and completely male individuals, but such individuals only rarely showed themselves inclined to my desires, I was often dependent on buying them for myself. However, since my desires are limited to persons of the lower classes, I always found those who could be had for money. I hope that the following frankness will not arouse your displeasure; I originally wanted to omit them, but for the sake of the completeness of this communication I must add them, since they should serve to enrich the casuistry.

I feel the need to perform the sexual act as follows:

[*LATIN: Taking the young man's penis into my mouth in such a way that by moving my mouth over it I might make the man I desire* cum, *I then spit out his seed onto the space between his genitals and his anus [perineum], order him to press his thighs together, and insert my penis against him and between his clenched thighs. While this is happening, the young man must embrace me as much as possible. The things that I said I had done before bring me the same pleasure just as if I, myself, am the one ejaculating. To reach ejaculation by inserting my penis into an anus or from receiving oral sex is not at all delightful to me. But I've found men who have received my penis and in doing the things that I described above have fully satisfied my lustful desires.*]

With regard to myself, I must mention the following: I am 186 cm tall, of completely masculine physical build, and, except for an abnormal irritability of the skin, healthy. I have very thick black hair on my head and a beard. My genitals are of medium size and of normal build. I am able to perform the sexual act described above four to six times within 24 hours without feeling fatigue. My lifestyle is very regular. I enjoy alcohol and tobacco very moderately. I play the piano quite well, and some small compositions of mine have met with much acclaim. I have recently finished a novel, which, as a first work, has received favourable reviews in my circles. It deals with several problems from the life of contra-sexuals.

With the large number of fellow sufferers I know personally, I was of course often in a position to make observations about various types of abnormalities; perhaps the following information will be of value to you.

The most abnormal thing I got to know was the habit preferred to all others of a gentleman from the outskirts of Berlin. He prefers boys with unwashed feet, which he licks fanatically. A gentleman in Leipzig behaves very similarly to this, [*LATIN: who must insert his tongue into an anus*], possibly and preferably uncleaned. In Paris there is a gentleman who forced one of my friends [*LATIN: to urinate into his mouth*]. Various people, as I am assured, come to such ecstasy at the sight of riding boots and military uniforms that they spontaneously ejaculate.

The degree to which some people feel themselves to be women, which is not the case with me, is exemplified by two personalities in Vienna in particular. They both have female names; one is a hairdresser who calls himself 'French Laura', the other is a former butcher called 'Selcher-Fanny'. Both of them never miss an opportunity during carnival to show themselves in female disguise, always very outré. In Hamburg there is a personality who some people believe to be a woman, because she always walks around her flat dressed as a woman, only leaving the house now and then, and always in the same clothes. This gentleman even wanted to pretend to be a godmother at a baptism and caused a huge scandal. Female vices, gossip, unreliability and weakness of character are the rule with such individuals.

I know of several cases of perverted sex, in which epilepsy and psychoses are present; hernias are conspicuously frequent. In practice, as I came to be recommended by friends, several persons with diseases of the anus applied to me. I saw two syphilitic and one local chancre, several fissures and am at present treating a gentleman with pointed condylomata [warts] of the anus, which forms a cauliflower-shaped tumour almost the size of a fist. I saw a case of primary affection of the soft palate in Vienna in a young man who attended masquerade balls dressed as a woman and there lured young men away. He then pretended to be having a period and managed it so that the others used him [*LATIN: orally*]. He is said to have lured 14 people in this way on one and the same evening. Since I have not found anything about the intercourse of pederasts in any of the publications on contra-sexualism that I have come across, I would like to conclude by telling you a few things about this.

As soon as contra-sexualists come to know each other, a detailed exchange of their previous experiences, loves and conquests takes place, as far as such a conversation is not excluded by the social differences of both. Only in very few cases does this conversation with new acquaintances not take place. The contra-sexualists call each other 'aunts', in Vienna 'sisters', and two very masculine-looking Viennese public prostitutes whom I met by chance and who were in a contra-sexual relationship with each other told me that the name 'uncle' is used for the corresponding appearance among women. Since I became aware of my abnormal drive, I have come into contact with well over a thousand like-minded people. Nearly every large town has some kind of meeting place and a so-called street. In smaller towns there are relatively few 'aunts', but in a town of 2300 inhabitants I found eight, in one of 7000 inhabitants eighteen, of whom I knew for certain, quite apart from those whom I suspected. In my hometown of about 30,000 inhabitants, I personally know about 120 'aunts'. Most of them, myself in particular to the highest degree, possess the ability to immediately judge another whether he is like them or not, as it is called in 'aunt language' 'reasonable or unreasonable'.[9] My acquaintances often marvel at how great the certainty of my eye is for this. I recognised seemingly all-male individuals as 'aunts' at first glance. On the other hand, I have the ability to behave in such a masculine manner that in circles to which I was recommended by acquaintances, doubts came to be raised about my 'authenticity'. When I am in the mood, I can behave completely like a woman.

Since most 'aunts', including myself, do not consider their abnormality to be a misfortune, but would regret it if this condition were to change, and since I and all others are convinced that the innate condition cannot be influenced, all our hopes are that the relevant paragraphs of the penal code will be amended to the effect that only rape or causing public nuisance, if these are simultaneously to be observed, should be considered a punishable offence.

3.8 NF (1890) Bb 3, 46–55

I am now in my thirty-sixth year. My father's family has always been considered a very healthy one. His father had married his own cousin. My mother, as I have heard, comes from very nervously agitated parents, but as far as I remember, was herself a very calm, highly educated woman, only nervous now and then and suffered quite often from headaches and pains in the spine. Her four sisters all suffer from migraines. The son of one of them was sent to an insane asylum several times after a failed suicide attempt and died there. My sister and one brother are quite normal in character; my eldest brother is completely a man of temper, of great sensitivity and completely lacking in energy. I suspect my third brother of being contra-sexual like me. I know for certain that he felt this way 10–11 years ago. Sometime later he told me that he didn't want to have anything to do with it, asked me to follow his example and from then on, I have had to suffer a lot from him morally, although the subject never came up between us directly. A year ago, I heard several times that he still felt the same way as before but was leading a quasi-marital life. I have not investigated further and do not want to hear anything more about it. So much for my relatives, and now it's my turn.

I was a very healthy, strong person, went through the childhood illnesses (measles etc.) quite normally and then always remained healthy until I was 18, when, as a result of a fall on my forehead, I went through a 14-day severe fever with headaches. I don't remember in which year I began to masturbate, but it must have started in my seventh year, perhaps earlier. Without seduction. Grown men—especially officers, my father's friends and performing riders—have always had a special attraction, and I often sought opportunities to be whipped by them. For lack of something better, I was also quite unruly on purpose at our boys' games, where some older boys always had to be present, so that I was sentenced to a beating, where I always tried to get my head between the legs of my executors, which, apart from the beating, aroused me even more. When I was five-and-a-half years of age, during a journey, we came to a ruin where a robber baron had once lived, and the guide knew the cruellest stories to tell about him. For a long time, I could not get this out of my mind, and I often thought of myself in the place of one of his victims; I often saw myself pressed between his thighs and my head pressed against his genitals, naturally imagining that I was going to be tortured by him in some way. I was always on the best of terms with our grooms; only the fear of discovery kept me from sexual acts, although it often consumed me like an inner fire. So I was content to let them touch me as roughly as possible, even to lie down in their beds or to watch and help them dress or undress. At one time my father (I was 10 or 11 years of age at the time) came to me with a slipper to slap me on my bottom, and on this occasion, instead of remorse, I got a violent erection and almost ejaculated. Moral sermons always had much better success. When I was eight-and-a-half years of age, I was seduced by a friend (of the same age) into mutual masturbation, and this relationship continued until I was 18 years of age. It is strange that love was completely absent, while at the same time I had intimate friendships and love relationships (purely platonic) with other friends. I have to say that these relationships would not have remained platonic if the people concerned had only encouraged me to go further. But they all had no idea of what was going on inside me. I usually had a special friend and during this time, that is, as long as I was allowed to socialise with him, all my other friends were of no importance to me. If he was then transferred to a school in another town, it always cost me a dull, lonely time, during which I withdrew from everything until I gradually felt affection for another of my fellow pupils again. During this time, the above-mentioned boy actually only served to satisfy my sexual desires; now I am extremely indifferent to him, whereas I still feel warm friendship for my platonic lovers, without any sexual desires. A year after the departure of my best, most beloved friend, I met a Dane. He was a courtier in a family in my father's town. I had seen him many times on the street and immediately fell in love with him; it was my first real love. I don't think it's possible for a normal man to love a woman more deeply or more hotly than I did at that time. Maybe I felt like a woman even then. I do not know. I would have given my life and everything for that man if he had asked me to. My friend had felt the same way as I did; he, too, had felt for me immediately. I still remember, as I do today, that the moment our eyes met for the first time, I felt a stab in my heart and had to hold onto the wall to keep from slurring my words. Arriving home in my room, I could only cry. You must forgive me this sojourn; I have only mentioned this story because I want to show that in our detested and frowned-upon class, the heart, that is, the whole inner man, comes to suffer just as much, perhaps even more, than in people of normal disposition. I will now be brief. This relationship lasted eight months and was interrupted when my friend left. It was the hottest love on both sides; we only kissed and hugged each other in the beginning, but later we started masturbating each other. We never spoke a word to each other about it. It came and went before we knew what was happening to us. We gave each other gifts of flowers, paintings and other small works, played music together a lot and were happy. During the last times we spent together, he often asked me to forgive him for having brought me this far, but I was well aware that I had always been born to do this, even though I had no idea of what I was to see in later years.

My friend became more and more melancholy as time went on; I suffered from it and then gradually fell into a similar mood. It came very close to being a double suicide instead of his departure.

After the separation, I spent the saddest months of my life, completely closed off, hardly even communicating with my father, who could not explain my condition. My brothers and sisters were all away from home by then.

Finally, on my twenty-first birthday, my father sent me to Paris. Even there, my grief for my lost friend, who was miserably eking out a living and whom I supported as best I could, continued. Perhaps also the awareness of the miserable situation of the other prevented me from returning to the joy of life. Finally, I could no longer bear the state of my soul. After I had repeatedly struggled with suicidal thoughts for days, even weeks, I wrote the unfortunate man off (I am still ashamed of myself today), and in this way I really did manage to feel a little lighter around the heart again. Now, however, the other struggle has become all the more important. In earlier years, I had not been able to understand why my friends (of the same age) were already attracted to the opposite sex, while I did not even feel the slightest stirring in myself. This gave me a lot of headaches, but I thought that this must come with time. In P., however, I thought it was high time, since I found several of my acquaintances, who were one or two years younger, already quite finished in their dealings with women: I often went to bars where the prostitutes met, always with the intention of accompanying one of them, but I could never bring myself to do so, since I completely lacked any excitement towards them. I always knew how to get away from joint expeditions to brothels by telling my acquaintances that such things disgusted me and that I could only go with one woman at a time. I did it like that for three months until I finally said to myself: it has to be done! I joined one of the prostitutes without feeling the slightest desire. The result was more than doubtful. During the evening I did not achieve an erection, felt deadly boredom, wished I was on top of the world, but stayed with the person in the hope of achieving a result. In the morning, with much difficulty, coitus succeeded. Without any pleasure, after endless time, and immediately after ejaculation being seized by repulsion and disgust, I got up and left. I could not get rid of the smell of this woman for days. No eau de cologne or perfume could help. It haunted me and was horrible to me. I always suffered from this disgusting addition even in my later attempts, while the smell of a man I liked was very pleasant to me. A few weeks later, in another serious attempt, I suffered a much more ignominious defeat. All it took was for the prostitute to lie in bed with me, undressed, and after I had tried in vain to achieve an erection, I had to get out again. I was seized with such horror that I could not have stayed for the world.

Even then, although I was only in contact with the woman for a few seconds, the smell haunted me. Then came a time of helplessness. I had no idea of the existence of urnings. I still believed myself to be all alone with my indefinable urge, despite my earlier relationship with a man (the one mentioned above). I must also mention that even while I was making those futile attempts with the opposite sex, many men had looked at me. Although I felt very sensually excited towards one or the other, I could not come to terms with my situation. For a short time, since I could no longer associate with women, nor even feel the slightest need to do so, I fell into a state of general agitation. Either sleepless nights, or if sleep ever came, I had the wildest dreams in which men played the leading role. In the spring I usually got up at three or four o'clock, even though I was dead tired, because I couldn't stay in bed any longer due to the excitement; then I would go for a walk for five or six hours, arrive exhausted at the office, where one of the employees would keep me busy in my thoughts all day. It was an agonising time, often interwoven with suicidal ideas. Whether I masturbated during that time, I don't remember, but I rather think it was not the case. One evening at a garden concert, I noticed that a gentleman looked at me very conspicuously every time I passed by, and I felt, as it were, magnetised, but I got through that evening still unplucked. We got lost in the crowd, but I couldn't stop thinking about the man and recognised him immediately the next time we met at the same concert. I can't say exactly whether I went to the pub at that time in the hope of meeting the gentleman again. In any case, his intention had become quite clear to me, and I still remember very clearly that at that time, I had the most definite feeling of an imminent crisis in my life. Suffice to say we met again after the concert. A little more isolated, the person in question spoke to me. We arranged to meet the next evening. I have seldom gone through such a struggle as I did on the day on which the rendezvous was to take place. Should I go? Should I not go? Yes? No? A hundred times I said to myself, 'No!', and until after dinner I stuck to 'No'. The next thing I knew, I was going. We met in the dark, and I was seized with an infinite rage, I slapped the gentleman hard across the face and told him he was a—Pig!—Then I walked up and away, thinking that now I was saved. From there, I went straight back to take advantage of the mood (for I had been in the greatest sensual excitement all day by thinking of the gentleman) and went to one of the places where the ladies make themselves amiable, with the intention of making another attempt. It was in vain; I had hardly seen all the women when all sensuality left me; I would not have been able to squeeze the hand of even one of them. No sooner had I arrived home than the old passion was loose again. Eight days had not passed before another gentleman noticed me at the same garden concert. He sat down next to me, began to bring the tips of his feet closer to mine and after a short time I knew where I stood. The man was neither young nor handsome; I don't know what attracted me to him that evening, but I gave myself to him. As a result, although I never actually came to love him, I did like him warmly. He initiated me into all the mysteries, and soon I knew (to the detriment of my seducer) that many young people whom I had particularly liked would be very glad of my acquaintance. That friend was also the first one to sodomise me, which, despite all the initial pain, gave me an undreamt-of sensation of lust. I must confess that even today, this type (passive sodomy) is the one that appeals to me the most. I believe I feel exactly what a woman feels during coitus. From then on, I never had intercourse with a person of the opposite sex in Paris. I suddenly found myself completely in my element and would never have felt any remorse about it had it not been for the fact that the general view of this topic, and later specifically my brother's moral sermons, had, so to speak, inoculated me against it.

I had to suffer a great deal for the consequences of my role as a woman in the sexual act, but when I was healthy again, I could not let go of it until today, although very long interruptions took place, as you can see from the following. Now a time of rapture began for me; my seducer had to return to his home country, so I used my freedom to make up for what I had missed for a long time, for I had a serious thirst for sexual intercourse. Perhaps I was so careless because I never found in any of them what I was really looking for, namely, a true friend worthy of me—the so-called aunts have always been repugnant to me and still are today. I only socialised with them as an exception, and only when one impressed me with his beauty for the moment. As soon as I noticed something feminine, something unmanly in their movements and manners, the whole attraction was over. Finally, just one year after my arrival in Paris, I met a gentleman for whom I immediately became passionate and to whom I gave myself completely. That was the best time of my life; we understood each other so completely, and, although we lived in different flats, we lived almost like husband and wife. This relationship, which I still think back to today with sincere longing (after 10 years), lasted until I had to leave Paris. However, we were often separated from each other due to my friend's travels. In the meantime, I passed my boredom with fleeting acquaintances, but in my mind, my friend was at the top of the list. At our respective reunions, we confessed to each other with full pardon and then loved each other all the more. I cannot imagine a happier love and friendship. I had to go home in the autumn of 1881. The first moral sermons by my brother, who had lived with me in Paris for two months, took place at this time. The effect was such that I began to believe that I was a wretch and an outcast after all. I visited various places but kept away from all men out of shyness. However, despite multiple sexual opportunities, I did not feel the slightest excitement towards women. In the year 1882 I went to London. There I again received letters from my brother, who reminded me of my past life and reproached me anew. Here, too, I tried to resist my urge for a while, but had two relapses, after which I felt great moral hangover each time I thought of my brother's letters. He also managed, without directly requesting it, that I cut off all correspondence with my dear Parisian friend as a result of his admonitions. But with that, all my joy was gone. Shall I confess to you that a few weeks ago I wrote to the same friend again! I also received a reply, and I am very happy to see that we have remained the same loyal friends despite the 10 years of total separation. It has been a long time since I was as happy as I was a few days ago when I received the letter. The first six months in London were very much like the first months in Paris. I kept away from men for the reasons I have just mentioned. Twice I managed coitus with women, but only with the utmost effort and by first having to help myself up with brandy and whisky. These times, too, I had not the slightest pleasure and longed with all my fibre for a man.

At last, I found one, neither handsome nor actually what I would have liked, very educated, but what particularly captivated me, very musical. I also lived with him for a year as if in a marriage; we got along very well, but gradually dissolved the intimate relationship and each went his own way. We are still very friendly with each other when we meet again after long intervals.

In this way, two years passed without me seeing much of other men. I then went to America to take up a position, wandered around there again for a long time without any friend—there I got used to masturbating again, I couldn't get used to women. Three attempts went very miserably without any trace of erection. In the end, I gave it up altogether so as not to attract the attention of the women in the brothels who frequented my acquaintances. I met a very handsome man there, of very good family, of rather limited intellect, but with excellent singing talent and voice and of an extremely friendly nature. He soon came to be my only friend, but only wanted to be loved platonically. He loved kissing and hugging very much, but he never became sexually excited. I even think he was quite indifferent to women too. He was a strict Catholic and advised me to convert in order to triumph over my own desires. I really did so eight months later. I studied the whole doctrine, conquered myself to the best of my ability and really reached a stage where I became rather indifferent to men. At that time, I would have loved to disappear into a convent forever with a sincere desire. Perhaps it would have been best for me, for what followed later did not serve to raise my morale. During that time, I also gave up onanism almost entirely. Occasionally once a month, the motive was merely to get rid of the horrible urge. When I fell, I reproached myself most bitterly for my weakness, but it happened again and again.

On the return journey to Europe, the ship's waiters immediately began to take a lively interest in me, but (due to shyness on my part) no interesting acquaintances were made. When I arrived in London, I immediately made a few street acquaintances, as well as in Belgium on my way through, but I did not enjoy it because of religious considerations. Then I spent another four months in Vienna, using all my energy without any sexual intercourse, in which my new religion undoubtedly supported me first and foremost. From there I went to Rio, and during the journey I made a male acquaintance who snared me again for the duration of the journey. When I arrived in Rio, I was able to refrain from acquaintances for another five to six months, but during that time I masturbated again when the urge became too strong. Even then, religion kept me on the right level. What turned me away from it were the numerous spicy stories you heard concerning the priests there, some glimpses behind the scenes of monastic life and so on. I do not want to excuse myself in any way, but these are the reasons that gave me back to manly love without barriers. The opportunity was rare, however, and the pleasure all the more precious for that reason. I got to know a man there, but he had such a dubious reputation in this respect that I could only visit him at night. We didn't know each other during the day. After him, two or three others. In 1887, I left the place to move to Java. There, unfortunately, I had no choice but to masturbate miserably, for I was never able to get used to the women there any more than to European women, despite the great need and lack of men. If I had wanted to, I could have found myself a compliant man every night, Chinese or Indian or Javanese, but I didn't dare because this would soon have come to light.

It is possible that I still had like-minded friends there, but they were all too uninteresting for me to seek out. In this way, I always felt excluded from the company of my colleagues, who must have noticed my total abstinence. Thank God they were too fond of me to ever make an embarrassing remark. I spent the last few years like a hermit, until fever and a weak heart drove me back to Europe in April of this year, probably without the possibility of returning to the tropics. My long journeys are the result of: (1) an innate urge to see the world, (2) quite specifically because in my father's town my perverse urge would have caused me unhappiness to the point of despair, and (3) because I (gifted with acknowledged musical talent) have never been able to decide to enter my father's dry monotonous office life. During the whole time, except for the last three-and-a-half years, I have only worked in offices, but the charm of the foreign country and the tropical environment has helped me to endure it all. For the last three years I have only been in the open air.

All that remains is to give you an idea of my outer person and character. I am 1.83 metre tall; as far as I can judge, I have a normal build; my hands and feet are large; the former have very long, thin fingers. Overall, I am not fat, but not skinny either. My muscles are quite prominent. Shape of face rather (narrow) oval, teeth in upper jaw almost all bad. Nose very prominent and curved upwards (but not bohemian). My eyes are considered beautiful, the expression of which has often been called rapturous, dreamy, also melancholic. Others might use the expression 'swimming' if I understood this term correctly. Moustache is not very luxuriant, but very soft and rather long-haired. Head hair quite luxuriant. My upper abdomen is almost completely hairless, but the lower parts of my thighs are well covered, as are my calves. Genitals are quite normally formed, but not very large. I think I look completely male, and very few of my companions notice my special features; only my eyes betray me here and there. I owe the majority of my 'conquests' to them. I, myself, can find nothing beautiful about me. In my family I am told that I am completely like my mother.

To this day, I have not been able to define my character. I used to think I knew myself, but since then I have come up against all kinds of contradictions. The melancholy temperament has prevailed for many years, probably as a result of the sins of youth, but in any case, largely as a result of the eternal compulsion to pretend and lie and hide myself. The letters that arrived from time to time from my brother, who, although he had no idea of my inner struggles, always knew how to reprimand me and bring up old things, also contributed to making me serious and withdrawn. I used to be very lively, learned easily, but was never a 'diligent' pupil, always in foreign parts of the world in my thoughts. Travelogues and pictures of overseas countries interested me the most. This preference still prevails today. In stark contrast to this, I have never had a taste for truly masculine sports. As a little boy, I loved to cook, could spend hours secretly doing my sister's dolls' hair, and loved to make women's costumes for my theatre figures until it came to me that I was forbidden to do so. In general, the theatre performances were more puppet shows than anything else. I also liked to dress in women's clothes and went to balls in such costumes several times. I could sew and knit quite well and can still help myself when I need something. Incidentally, I have never put on women's clothes for 11 years and will never do so again. On the contrary, I try to appear as masculine as possible in all my doings and activities. I do take a lot of care with my grooming, in that I always dress in English modern clothes, but never excessively or ostentatiously. I would very much like to wear jewellery but do so only in a very limited way so as not to attract attention.

Riding, hunting, fencing and so on interest me very little, but I enjoy walking very much; mountain tours have always been a pleasure for me. Reading newspapers and politics are about the most repugnant things I know. My hobbies are first and foremost music, and secondly painting. If my father had allowed it, I would undoubtedly have become a pianist, and I am convinced that I would have gone very far; that would have been the only occupation for which I would never have lost stamina. It is generally said that I have a very beautiful approach and soulful performance, although I lack fluency. I also have a great sense for interior decoration, but not for the conventional, fashionable, but for tasteful, completely unconstrained styles, possibly with palm trees and many flowers. In paintings, I am particularly attracted to beautiful, noble landscapes with distant views à la Claude Lorrain.

In real life I have the same tastes; I love nature, I love living in the mountains or by the ocean. I also never tire of being at sea. I keep very little company; I prefer to be alone than in the company of people who are indifferent to me. I always feel the partition that separates me from others, and the gentlemen whose acquaintance I make here and there for social reasons do not come to intimacy either. Larger festivities, at which others can get into the most joyful mood, have a downright depressing effect on me, without my knowing why. I like to socialise with women if they are intellectually stimulating, even elegant, but as soon as the slightest inkling of sexual contact appears even remotely, I have to avoid them, otherwise I become quite awkward. All last summer ladies tried to make my acquaintance, but I had to give them up because I could smell the taint from afar. I have already received gentle hints from home that the time has come for me to marry, but I will never be able to be won over by this, as I have the firmest conviction that I could only make a woman unhappy. Besides, it would be dreadful for me to bind myself firmly to a woman, even if I had the certainty that I would not have to have sexual intercourse at all. I would much rather marry my friend in Paris, if that were possible.

I only feel really in my element and satisfied with a person from my social class, a real man, good-looking, with the same talents as I, with a good appearance, and with whom the sensual moment has already receded into the background. I am ashamed to say, but for the sake of truth it must be said: an ugly, uninteresting-looking person, even if he is of good character and also like-minded, will never achieve the same degree of intimacy with me. I have always disliked pronounced urnings, that is, those whose movements, speech and so on show the slightest hint of femininity. I only associated with them for a short time. The few close acquaintances I have kept are all men.

I cannot in the least find that my condition seems unnatural, for as far back as I can remember, I have always felt the same way. It is rather in my occasional attempts with women that I have found it something, if not unnatural, at least very unpleasant and unsatisfactory. I have morally endured much, very much, but not because I recognised my impulse as morbid, but because of the general contempt which strikes us from all sides. When I often heard people talk about this subject, I could never master a feeling of bitterness, because I said to myself, 'You were born that way and you will remain that way forever!' and then I got angry at the senseless expressions that blindly condemn without lifting a finger to learn the truth about us. The only thing that depresses me is that I cannot get rid of onanism, and although it is abhorrent to me, I want to get beyond that. That the other special anomaly will ever come to an end, I have no hope of that, but would gladly, if I had the opportunity, subject myself to an attempt. Your work *Psychopathia Sexualis* has brought me much comfort; it contains passages which I could have copied, so much are they unconsciously taken from my own life. Since I saw your benevolent interest in our disreputable class in it, my heart has become much lighter; until now I had heard only condemnation from all sides; this was the first time I encountered someone who showed me that we are not quite as bad as we are made out to be, and even though I do not consider myself blameless, I feel a great burden lifted from me anyway.

I, for my part, have no hope of experiencing a change for the better for us. That will come to us later. Even if we are to be treated more leniently by the courts in the future (I have never come into conflict with them, thank God, and without being called upon to do so), who will abolish the prejudice that has existed against us in society since time immemorial? As long as this exists, our moral sufferings will not come to an end.

3.9 NF (1890) Bb 8, 59–61

I was born in 1856. My mother had given birth to two boys before me and, when she was in blessed circumstances with me for the third time, had the ardent wish to give birth to a girl. A few years before her death, my mother was highly hysterical; her condition improved; a short time later, however, she acquired a fatal illness (breast cancer) and died in great agony. My father was extremely nervous, morbidly sensitive and irritable and died three years ago after a short illness, an internal malignant abscess. My upbringing was completely misguided, mollycoddled. I must have practised masturbation in my earliest youth, perhaps in my seventh or eighth year. The manner of self-abuse was peculiar and deviated from the usual form. In my fourteenth year, as a result of admonitions and remorse, I stopped and only fell into the old bad habit three or four times from that time on. I was already a very nervous child in my early youth; in my fifteenth year I suffered from melancholy and had all kinds of neurasthenic and hysterical states. This epoch, however, lasted only half a year, and I was relatively well for some years.

During this period, I discovered (after, by the way, inclinations and signs had already been present in boyhood), at first with rather naive and careless astonishment, later with growing uneasiness, and at last (after I was perfectly clear about it) with the utmost dismay, that my sexual inclinations were abnormal both physically and psychically. I always found the female unattractive, her sexual advances nauseating, and was receptive to the male touch to the opposite extent. My older brothers and other friends, however, described pederasty to me as such an abominable crime that I avoided sexual intercourse with another man out of fear until I was 23. This abstinence, however, did not prevent my nerves from undergoing another highly embarrassing crisis until shortly before my 'fall'. From the age of 17–23 I suffered greatly from pollutions, which caused the greatest tension.

Unfortunately, I already showed great talent for music in my early youth; I became a musician, and this occupation naturally contributed to a great extent to completely shattering my nerves.

At the age mentioned, I made the acquaintance of a handsome young man who gave me my first introduction to direct sexual contact; I could not resist his powerful charms and had to give way to temptation. He gave me the most reassuring information about the consequences that I had dreadfully imagined, and he not only succeeded in making my misgivings disappear, but I also found this new period of my life attractive and tempting, and during this time, when I did, however, practise sexual intercourse in a rather modified way, I felt relatively better than before.

During this time, my talent reached artistic maturity, and I successfully went on many concert tours through most European countries. These, as well as the constant change of air, had a beneficial effect on my physical and mental condition, and I never had more joy in life than at this time. At the same time, I made numerous acquaintances with 'like-minded people'. I took as lovers French counts and dukes, German soldiers, Swedish peasants, grooms, elegant officers, English lords, Spanish marquis, Hungarian magnates, artists, scholars, celebrities (whom everyone should know by name), but also the most vulgar fellows; my taste was (unlike most of 'we others') not exclusive, in no particular direction; I took everything that chance brought me. Of all those who more or less captivated my mind, only one was able to win my heart completely. It was a young Frenchman, beautiful in body and soul; I have known him for almost 10 years now, and he has had the most powerful influence on me from that time to this day. Passionately in love with him for the first few years, I went through all the delights and torments of that stage; today it has been replaced by the deepest love of friendship, capable of the greatest mutual sacrifice and self-denial. I have never known a more ideal relationship, neither between woman and man, nor in the numerous 'other menages'.

Finally, I want to say that I do not consider it a great misfortune, either for myself or for others who have contra-sexual feelings. We come to be amply compensated for the disadvantages that arise for us (not tolerating social laws, and therefore eternal lies and dissimulation) by the mysterious, enchanting charm that the matter offers. Besides, we come to be much more spared in regard to contagious diseases and expenditure of money. With only half caution and sensible moderation, we risk relatively little. Those who come into contact with the police and are brought to justice are mostly to blame themselves through carelessness or their own foolishness. It would be high time, by the way, in our otherwise so enlightened and sensible age, to provide these millions of persons, whom nature has played a trick on and who are in fact completely innocent of it, with some kind of justice in this respect. In public, all impropriety is forbidden; but what two people do behind their own four walls with mutual consent without harming a third person that should not be forbidden by human laws.

May this epilogue of my own recorded confessions serve as a small contribution to the salvation of many outlaws.

In conclusion, I take the liberty of expressing the opinion about this topic, that I do not consider contrary sexual feelings to be nervous diseases. As miserable and ill as I feel, I must nevertheless state that I know many, many people with the same feelings who are in perfect health and have nerves of steel.

3.10 NF (1891) Bb 12, 127–31

R: *PS7 (1892) Bb 122, PS8 (1893) Bb 122*

I am writing down my tale of woe as best I can, guided solely by the desire to use this autobiography to help shed a little light on the misunderstanding and cruel misconceptions about 'contrary sexual feeling' that unfortunately still prevail in so many circles.

I am 37 years of age and come from parents who were both very nervous. I only mention this because the thought has often crossed my mind that my contra-sexual feeling came about by way of heredity; but this assertion is only a very vague one. Of my grandparents, whom I did not know, I would only like to mention as remarkable that my maternal grandfather was known as the great Don Juan.

I was a rather weak child and suffered greatly from so-called gout in the first two years of my life. As a result, my comprehension and memory may also have suffered, since I learn things that do not interest me only slowly and with difficulty and easily forget what I have learned. I would also like to mention that before I was born, my mother was subjected to violent mental upheavals and is said to have been frightened very often. From the age of three I have been completely healthy and, so far, have been spared any major illnesses. Only when I was a boy of 12–16 years did I sometimes have very strange, indescribable nerve sensations, which were particularly noticeable in my head and fingertips, and which made me feel as if my whole being wanted to dissolve. For many years now, however, the episodes have not occurred at all. Otherwise, I am a rather strong man with abundant hair growth and a thoroughly masculine nature.

Already at the age of six I independently turned to masturbation, to which I was unfortunately quite violently addicted until I was 19 years of age, and to which I still frequently resort, for lack of something better, although I recognise the reprehensibility of this passion and also feel quite weakened every time, whereas sexual intercourse with a man does not affect me in the least, but on the contrary gives me a feeling of being strong. At the age of seven I began to attend school and soon felt a strong liking for some of my classmates, but I made nothing more of it. At grammar school, at the age of 14, I came to learn from my classmates about the sexual life of human beings, which had been completely unknown to me until then, but without taking much interest in the matter. At that time, I was also engaged in mutual masturbation with two or three friends, into which they had seduced me, and which had an enormous appeal for me. I was still not aware of the perversity of my sex drive, but considered my offences to be youthful sins, as they would come to be committed by all boys of that age. Interest in the female sex, I thought, would come to me in time. So, I reached the age of 19. During the following years I was madly in love three times, once with a very beautiful actor, then with a bank clerk and one of my friends, the latter two of whom were nothing less than beautiful, sensually captivating people, but which love was only a purely platonic one that occasionally degenerated into fervent poems. It was perhaps the most beautiful time of my life, when I looked at everything with pure innocent eyes, but in my twenty-first year I began to notice that I was not quite like my friends, since I felt no pleasure at all in male pursuits, took little pleasure in smoking, drinking and playing cards, and was truly deathly afraid of brothels. I never went to a brothel, because I always managed to steal away under some pretext. I now began to think about myself; I often felt terribly abandoned, miserable and unhappy and longed for a friend with the same disposition, but without thinking that there could be other people like me. At the age of 22, I met a young person who finally enlightened me about the contra-sexual feeling and those associated with it, because he, also an urning, was in love with me. The scales fell from my eyes, and I bless the day that brought me this enlightenment. From then on, I looked at the world with completely different eyes, saw how many people like me had the same fate, and began to learn to come to terms with this fate as best I could.

Unfortunately, things went very badly, and I am often still gripped by a doggedness and a deep hatred of the modern institutions that treat us poor urnings in a terribly stepmotherly manner. For what is our lot? In most cases we are not understood, we are ridiculed and despised, and when things are going well and in a few rare cases we are understood, we are pitied like poor sick or insane people—and pity has always made me sick. I now began to play the comic in order to deceive my fellow men about my inner life, and it gave me great satisfaction every time I succeeded. I also got to know several companions of fate with whom I established relationships, but unfortunately, they were always short-lived, as I was very timid and cautious, but also very choosy and spoiled.

I have always completely abhorred sodomy as something unworthy of human beings, and I only wish that all my fated friends would do the same; unfortunately, this is not the case with so many, for if everyone thought about it in the same way as I do, the contempt and ridicule of people who feel differently would come upon us even more unfairly than it has so far.

Towards the man I love, I feel completely like a woman, which is why I also behave rather passively during the sexual act. In general, my whole sensibility and feeling is feminine; I am vain, coquettish, addicted to cleaning and pleasing myself, love to dress beautifully and, in cases where I want to please, even resort to grooming arts, in which I am quite proficient.

As little as I am interested in politics, I am equally passionate about music and am an enthusiastic devotee of Richard Wagner, a preference I have noticed in most of us; I find that this music is so much in keeping with our nature.

I play the violin quite well, like to read a lot, but otherwise I have little interest in anything else; just as I am indifferent to everything else in life as a result of the deep resignation that is taking hold of me more and more.

Although I would have reason to be satisfied with my fate, since I live in a secure position as an engineer in a large German city, I take no pleasure in my profession. I would prefer to be completely independent and free to travel to lovely places with a beloved and otherwise be able to spend time with music and literature, especially at the theatre, which seems to me to be one of the greatest pleasures. To be the director of a court theatre would be most agreeable.

The only position or profession that really seems desirable to me is that of a great artist, be it singer, actor, painter or sculptor, whatever; and there is nothing more pleasing to me than the thought of being born on a royal throne, a wish that corresponds to my pronounced desire to rule. (If there really is a transmigration of souls, a subject with which I occupy myself a great deal and which seems very plausible to me, then I must have lived at some time as an emperor or some other ruler). But you have to be born to do all that, and since I am not, I lack the ambition for so-called social honours and awards.

As far as my tastes are concerned, I must mention an unfortunate dichotomy in them. Beautiful, intellectually very gifted young men of at least 20 years of age, who must be socially on the same level as I, seem to me to be made for a more platonic love, but I am completely content with a sincere but very ideal friendship that rarely goes beyond a few kisses. Sensually, however, I can only be attracted to rougher and stronger men who are at least as old as I am and who must be mentally and socially below me. The reason for this strange phenomenon may be that my rather strong sense of shame and my innate fearfulness and reserve have an inhibiting effect on men like me, so that in these cases I can only with difficulty and rarely achieve sexual excitement. That I suffer greatly from this dichotomy is explicable, since I am always afraid to reveal myself to these simple people beneath me, who are often available for money. I imagine nothing more terrible than a scandal that would immediately drive me to suicide. For I cannot imagine anything more horrifying than to suddenly be branded before the whole world by a minor carelessness or malice on the part of a first-class person from high society, and actually not being able to do anything about it. For what we do is nothing other than what all other normally disposed people are allowed to do at least as often, without being dishonoured and without shame; but the fact that we do not feel the same way as the great masses is not our fault, but a cruel game of nature.

Countless times I have racked my brain as to whether science, and within it a few free and unprejudiced thinking men, could not devise a means of providing us stepchildren of nature with a more tolerable position before the law and men. But each time I came to the same sad conclusion, that one must first know and be able to explain exactly a matter for which one is taking a stand. And who, up to the present day, has been able to precisely explain and define the contra-sexual feeling? And yet there must be some right explanation for it, some way by which the great multitude can be taught a milder and more reasonable judgment of it, above all the one thing at least, that one does not regard contra-sexual feeling as synonymous with pederasty, as is unfortunately done by most, I should like to say by all. By such a deed one would set up an indelible monument in the gratitude of thousands of living and future people, for urnings have existed, exist and will come to exist at all times and in greater numbers than one might suppose.

In Wilbrand's book, *Fridolins heimliche Ehe* (Fridolin's secret marriage),[10] I find a quite acceptable theory on this subject, since I, myself, have repeatedly had the opportunity to observe that not all urnings are equally man-loving, but that there are innumerable subdivisions, from the most effeminate man to the contra-sexual man, who just as often and gladly falls for female charms. This may also explain the so-called difference between innate and acquired contra-sexual sensation, which, in my inferior opinion, does not exist at all. However, I have encountered the same temperament, disposition and character traits in all 55 individuals whom I have met in the three years since my enlightenment on this subject; almost all of them are more or less idealists, smoke little or not at all, are bigoted, vain, addicted to pleasure and superstitious and generally combine (I must unfortunately confess) more the faults and dark sides of both sexes than their good qualities. I feel a true horror towards women in their sexual role, which I would never succeed in overcoming even with the use of all my extremely vivid imagination; nor have I ever tried, because I am completely convinced of the fruitlessness of such an attempt, which seems to me unnatural and sinful.

In purely social and friendly relationships I like to socialise with women and girls and am also a welcome companion in ladies' circles, as I am very interested in ladies' fashions and know how to talk about such things with great skill. I can be very cheerful and amiable when I want to be, but this gift of mine for conversation is mostly just comedy, which always tires me out and negatively affects me. I have always shown a great talent and interest in female work; as a child up to the age of 13 I loved to play with dolls, sewing their clothes myself, and even now it gives me great pleasure to make beautiful embroideries, which unfortunately I can only do in secret. I am just as fond of knick-knacks, photographs, flowers, sweets, toiletries and all kinds of trinkets, and my room, which I have furnished and decorated all by myself, resembles the rather overloaded boudoir of a lady.

As a special curiosity, I would like to mention that I have never suffered from wet dreams. I dream a lot and very vividly, almost every night, and occasional lascivious dreams only involve male figures, but I always wake up from them before ejaculation occurs. Actually, I am not very needy sexually, and I have periods of four to six weeks when the sexual urge almost does not assert itself at all. Unfortunately, these are rare and are usually followed by a more violent awakening of this so powerful instinct, which, if it is not satisfied, causes me severe physical and mental complaints. I then become ill-tempered, moody, sensitive, irritable and shy of people, but these qualities disappear again at the first best opportunity I have to satisfy my sexual instinct. In general, I must mention that my mood can change several times a day on the most trivial of occasions; it is like the weather in April.

I dance well and with pleasure, but I love dancing only for its rhythmic movement and because of my preference for music.

Finally, I would like to mention something that always arouses my displeasure. We are generally thought to be ill, and that is completely untrue. For every disease there is a remedy or palliative, and no power in the world can take away an urning's perverted natural disposition. Even suggestion, applied with much apparent success, cannot produce any lasting change in the soul-life of an urning. We confuse effect and cause. We are thought to be ill because most of us really become ill in time. I am firmly convinced that two-thirds of us have some kind of mental defect at a later age, if we reach it at all, and this is only too easy to explain. After all, what willpower and what nerves are needed to keep on pretending, lying and deceiving throughout one's life. How often does one have to join in the vituperations and invectives in the circle of normal people, when by chance the subject of contra-sexual feelings comes up, while each of these words wounds one to the core. On the other hand, to have to listen to the boring and indecent jokes and conversations about women and so on, which are commonplace in so-called good society nowadays, and to feign interest in and pay attention to them! To see so many beautiful male figures every day, every hour, to whom one cannot reveal oneself, often for weeks and months to have to do without the friend whose intercourse we need so much, and on top of that this terrible constant fear of betraying oneself before men and then standing there covered with shame and disgrace. It is really any wonder that most of us are incapable of any serious professional work, for we need all our willpower and endurance in the struggle with our sad fate. How damaging to our nerves to have to keep all our thoughts and feelings bottled up inside, where our already vivid imagination, nourished by all this, works all the more restlessly, so that we carry around a constant source of fire that only too often threatens to consume us. Happy are those of us who never fail to have the strength to carry on such a life, but happy also are those who have already overcome it.

Notes

1. This correspondent was almost certainly referring to Ulrichs' suggestion that urnings should be able to marry each other. His fourth pamphlet *Ara Spei* had been an early advocate of same-sex marriage when he asked why the bond of love between an urning and his (dioning) lover should not be recognised as equivalent to dioning marriages (Karl Heinrich Ulrichs, *Ara Spei*. Leipzig: H. Matthes, 1865. Trans. Lombardi-Nash as 'Book Five: Ara Spei' in *The Riddle of 'Man-Manly' Love*, vol. 1, §41–66, 207–16.) Later, in his tenth pamphlet *Prometheus*, after a Catholic dioning claimed that 'It just would not be possible to join two urnings or a dioning and urning in marriage' Ulrichs replied 'Why not? Why should Uranian love not have the right to step before the altar of God, who created it?' (Karl Heinrich Ulrichs, *Prometheus*. Leipzig: A. Serbe, 1870. Trans. Lombardi-Nash as 'Book Ten: Prometheus' in *The Riddle of 'Man-Manly' Love*, vol. 2, §32,

563.) Krafft-Ebing later credited the commitment to marriage-like relationship types as a convincing proof of moral seriousness: 'A more striking proof of the depth and sincerity of such a sexual sentiment on the part of numerous fellow citizens who are to be taken seriously and who feel themselves to be martyrs of their organisation and of social conditions could not be provided'. (Richard von Krafft-Ebing, 'Neue Forschungen auf dem Gebiet der Psychopathia Sexualis', *Jahrbuch für sexuelle Zwischenstufen* 3 (1901): 2.).

2. Hypospadias is a birth defect where the opening of the urethra is not at the tip of the penis.
3. Uncertain what is meant here. 'Esprit faux' (literally 'false spirit') could mean that he is a deceitful, manipulative or secretive person but the passage that follows makes it sound like he is talking about compulsive and disordered thinking.
4. This is a curious misapprehension that may relate to hypersexuality as a symptom of rabies.
5. Numa Numantius was the pseudonym used by Karl Heinrich Ulrichs in his first five pamphlets.
6. Christian Johann Heinrich Heine (1797–1856) was a renowned German poet, writer and literary critic.
7. Joseph Victor von Scheffel (1826–1886) was a German poet and novelist.
8. This is probably referring to the decision of the Reichsgericht (German Supreme Court) in Leipzig in 1878 to reclassify Paragraph 175 to cover all acts imitative of intercourse—that is, that used thrusting actions (anal, oral and interfemoral sex)—where mutual masturbation was notably not included as an illegal act.
9. According to one of Ulrichs's correspondents, quoted in the second edition of *Memnon*, 'vernünftig' (reasonable) was used as a vernacular term for urning. Karl Heinrich Ulrichs, *Memnon, Abtheilung II*. Schleiz: C. Hübscher'sche Buchhandlung, 1868. Translated by Michael Lombardi-Nash as 'Book Seven: Memnon II' in The *Riddle of 'Man-Manly' Love: The Pioneering Work on Male Homosexuality*, vol. 2 (Buffalo: Prometheus Books, 1994), 494n21; Letter 151 in Douglas Pretsell, *The Correspondence of Karl Heinrich Ulrichs, 1846–1894* (Cham: Palgrave Macmillan, 2020), 195.
10. Adolf von Wilbrandt (1837–1911) published *Fridolins heimliche Ehe* in 1875. This was the earliest novel on a homosexual subject in the German language.

CHAPTER 4

Two Polemics

4.1 PS4 (1889), 216–9

R: *PS5 (1890), 276–9*

You have no idea what a continuing struggle we all—and the thoughtful and sensitive among us most of all—still have to endure today and how much we have to suffer from the still prevailing false view of ourselves and our so-called immorality.

Your view that the phenomenon in question, as the final cause in most cases, is to be ascribed to an innate 'pathological' disposition will perhaps make it most possible to overcome the existing prejudices and, instead of disgust and contempt, to arouse compassion for us poor 'sick' people.

So, as much as I believe that the view you hold is one that is as beneficial as possible for us, in the interest of science I am not able to accept the word 'pathological' so readily and would like to take the liberty of giving you a few more arguments relating to it.

The phenomenon is abnormal under all circumstances, but the word pathological has another meaning which I cannot find applicable in this case, at least not in very many cases which I have had the opportunity to observe. I will admit beforehand that cases of mental disturbances, of nervous over-stimulation and so on can be found in a far higher proportion among the urnings than among other normal people. But is this increased

D. Pretsell, *Queer Voices in the Works of Richard von Krafft-Ebing, 1883–1901*, Genders and Sexualities in History,
https://doi.org/10.1007/978-3-031-17331-8_4

nervousness necessarily connected with the nature of being an urning, or is it not in the great majority of cases due to the fact that, as a result of the prevailing legislation and social prejudices, the urning cannot, like other people, easily and simply satisfy his innate sexual inclination?

The uranian youth, when he feels his first sexual impulses and naively expresses them to his friends, soon finds out that he will not find understanding with others; he now closes himself off. If he even informs a teacher or his parents of what moves him, the impulse, which is as natural to him as swimming is to a fish, is portrayed as depraved and sinful, and he is preached that it must be fought and suppressed at all costs. An inner struggle now begins, a violent suppression of the sexual impulse, and the more the natural satisfaction of it is suppressed, the more vividly the imagination begins to work and conjures up again and again the very images one would like to banish. The more energetically the person who fights this inner battle, the more the whole nervous system must suffer. Such a violent suppression of a drive that is so deeply implanted in us only develops the pathological phenomena that we can observe in many urnings, but it is not necessarily connected with the respective uranian disposition itself.

Some continue this constant inner struggle for a greater or lesser length of time and wear themselves out in the process; others finally come to the realisation that their innate, powerful drive cannot possibly be sinful, so they no longer attempt the impossible—the suppression of it. But now the series of suffering and constant agitation begins! The dioning,[1] when he seeks satisfaction for his sexual impulses, always knows how to find it easily; not so the urning! He sees the men who excite him, but he is not allowed to say anything, not even to let them know what moves him. He thinks that he alone in the whole world has such abnormal sensations. Naturally, he seeks contact with young men, but does not dare to confide in them. So, as a substitute, he resorts to giving himself the satisfaction he cannot otherwise achieve. Masturbation is practised on a large scale, and all the consequences of this vice become apparent. If then, after a certain time, a breakdown of the nervous system occurs, the pathological phenomenon is again not caused by being an urning in itself, but only by the fact that the urning, as a result of today's generally prevailing views, could not find the natural normal satisfaction of his sexual instinct and thus fell into masturbation.

Or let us now suppose that the urning had the rare good fortune of soon finding a soul with the same feelings, or that he had soon been enlightened by an experienced friend about what was going on in the urning world, he might be spared many an inner struggle, but a long series of excitation, worries and anxieties would also follow him at every step. Now he knows that he is no longer the only one in the world with such abnormal feelings; he opens his eyes and is surprised at how many associates he finds in all social circles and in all occupational classes; he also learns that there is prostitution among urnings as well as among dionings and that men-for-pay are to be had as well as strumpets. So there is no longer a lack of opportunities for the satisfaction of sexual urges. But how differently things develop here from the dionings!

Let us assume the happiest case. The sympathetic friend for whom one has longed all one's life has been found. But one must not openly show affection to him, as the young man does to the girl he loves. In constant fear, both must always conceal their relationship; even too great intimacy, which could easily arouse suspicion—especially if both are not of the same age or do not belong to the same social class—must remain hidden from the outside world. Thus, a chain of agitation begins with the relationship itself, and the fear that the secret could be betrayed or guessed at does not allow the poor man to enjoy himself. An occurrence that is indifferent to everyone else makes him tremble because it could arouse suspicion, and his secret could come to light, which would undermine his whole social position, and he would lose his office and profession. And this constant excitation, this perpetual fear and anxiety should pass without a trace and not have a repercussion on the whole nervous system?

Another, less fortunate, did not find a like-minded friend, but fell into the hands of a handsome man who at first willingly accommodated him until the innermost secrets were revealed to him. Now the most ingenious blackmail is practised. The unhappily persecuted man, faced with the alternative of paying or becoming a social pariah, of losing a respected position, of seeing disgrace befall him and his family, pays, and the more he pays, the greedier becomes the vampire who sucks at him, until finally only the choice remains between total financial ruin or dishonour. Who would be surprised if the nerves of each one was not up to this terrible struggle!

One person's nerves fail completely, a mental disorder sets in and the poor man finally finds peace in an insane asylum that he could not find in life. Another, in despair, puts an end to this unbearable state by committing suicide. How many of the often-inexplicable suicides of young men can be counted here is impossible to fathom! I do not think I am wrong when I say that at least half of the suicides among young men are due to such circumstances. Even in cases where it is not the ruthless blackmailer who pursues an urning, but only a relationship between two men which in itself is satisfactory, the discovery, or even the fear of discovery, often leads to suicide. How many officers who have had a relationship with one of their subordinates, how many soldiers who have had a relationship with a fellow soldier, have tried to escape the disgrace threatening them by taking a bullet the moment they thought they had been discovered! And similarly in all other professions!

If, therefore, it must certainly be admitted that more mental abnormalities and probably also more real mental disorders can be observed in urnings than in other people, this does not, however, prove that these mental disorders are necessarily connected with the urning nature and that one causes the other. It is my firm conviction that by far the greater part of the mental disorders or pathological dispositions observed in urnings are not to be put down to their sexual abnormality but are caused by the present wrong view of the urning nature and, in connection with this, by the existing legislation and the prevailing opinion on this subject. Whoever has the slightest idea of the abundance of mental and moral suffering, of the anxiety and worry which an urning must endure, of the eternal hypocrisy and subterfuge which he must employ in order to conceal his inherent urges, of the infinite difficulties which oppose the natural satisfaction of his sexual urges can only be surprised that more serious mental disorders and nervous diseases do not occur among urnings. Most of these pathological conditions would certainly not develop if the urning, like the dioning, could find sexual satisfaction in a simple and easy way, if he were not exposed to this eternal torturing anxiety!

4.2 FB (1891), 385–400[2]

I have passed the age of 45 and hold a higher post in the civil service. Recognising my sexual particularity and its 'social impossibility' early on, I decided at a young age to resign, accept my fate and take up the struggle with life in other areas. I wanted to at least achieve prestige and influence in this world that was hostile to me.

Constant striving, some talent and even more fortunate side circumstances have provided me with an outwardly enviable position in life and, without compensating me for the deprivation of that good in which H. Drummond sees 'the greatest thing in the world', have at least helped to distract me from myself to a certain extent, to protect me so far from discouragement and to make my fate bearable. But now to my 'medical history'.

My ancestors were almost without exception civil servants or farmers through a number of generations. I know of no mental or remarkable physical ailments in my family. On the contrary, physical fitness and mental vigour up to a ripe old age are native to my family. I have not noticed any sexual peculiarities among my relatives. I am unmarried. My outer appearance is hardly conspicuous. I have always enjoyed physical exercise, even outside my profession, and have therefore not been unsuccessful. I like to smoke, but without passion, and I am abstinent in the consumption of alcoholic beverages. My state of health could not be better, neither physically nor mentally.

The peculiarity of my sexual constitution is that my inclination is predominantly, but not exclusively, towards my own sex. It corresponds to a predominant sexual aversion or at least indifference towards the opposite sex. This relationship or disproportion has persisted unchanged since the faintest beginnings of my sexual life. Even as a child, I rapturously loved young boys and older boys. As a boy I suffered from paroxysms of friendship. What I thought was friendship was, as I later realised, something else. But this something else rested in the purest innocence until I was 16. Then it happened, during a stay in the country, that I stretched out over a beautiful boy lying on his back on the ground during a scuffle with this friend of my age; a hitherto unknown feeling of lust seized me, transformed the wrestling with an opponent into an impetuous embrace, and I was surprised at the moment of greatest excitement by an ejaculation—the first and scanty one. I kept my experience a secret from everyone and repeatedly sought and found the same pleasure, though not too often. At the same time, I surrendered to masturbation, which I had also discovered myself around the same time, but curtailed this practice again a year later, after a medical book I had obtained by chance had instilled in me a vivid disgust for it. The reading of this book also induced me to curb the impulses of sexual desire in me, to which a religious and strict moral upbringing, but most of all frequent nocturnal pollutions, which alarmed me for years, may have contributed. The latter were very predominantly provoked by male dream stimuli, rarely—in a ratio of about 1 to 50—by female dream stimuli, and this is how it has remained to this day. Likewise, only in very isolated cases have female persons of pleasing appearance interested me sexually; under correspondingly favourable circumstances I have even reached coitus a few times and, in my opinion, with normal success and satisfaction. My drive for my own sex, on the other hand, is much more general and much more intense at the same time. It is aroused to a greater or lesser extent by every young man who sprouts fuzz on his lips, if he is not deformed. The sight of a beautiful youth, however, seems to subordinate the sensual element of my sexual feeling to a higher spiritualised pathos and seizes me to the inmost depths of my heart. The satisfaction of the longing awakened by this, the intimate intercourse with the object of it, would give me the highest bliss; I would be able to grant him anything and sacrifice everything for him.

Even when such a desire of my heart has not been granted, even when I have renounced the sensual satisfaction appropriate to my nature, and even when my share in the pleasures of life has thus been reduced to that of the simplest labourer, I have nevertheless been anxious, within the admittedly very constricting barriers drawn for me by my firm resolution and the shyness to compromise my extremely favourable social position in all other relationships, to shed some light on my life path in favour of my sexual feelings as well. I have felt more at ease in my interactions with my subordinates than they even suspected, since they only sensed the benevolence from my secret affection and idolised their superiors. What has been communicated here will already sufficiently reveal a special nuance of the 'contrary sexual feeling' in my condition. It is thoroughly original and predominantly, but not exclusively, homosexual. But what caprice could there be that could not be entrusted to nature!

Whether homosexuality, be it total or partial, is to be considered pathological even if it is original, is a question I, as a layman, must leave open. As testimony for the opposite, I can only refer to my other subjective well-being. In any case, the abnormal should not necessarily be identifiable with the pathological, otherwise a far more pathological phenomenon would have to be seen in the psyche of a Rafael or Mozart in relation to that of the normal average person than in the urning in relation to the normal sexual.

I can be excused for saying in what way I satisfy my very lively sexual sensual needs. Society is responsible for forcing decent men to indulge in unnatural shamelessness. However, I do not feel any health disadvantages from it, thanks to the moderation dictated by an understandable reluctance and health concerns. I am also of the opinion, by the way, that 'masturbation' in combination with homosexuality is in any case less harmful than when it is practised with a normal sexual disposition. The harmfulness of the unnatural, arbitrary discharge of semen is probably mainly due to the fact that the mechanical peripheral stimulus alone is effective. Where, on the other hand, the sexual stimulus emanates from the centre, the otherwise abnormal satisfaction is at least approximated to the normal one. The homosexual, however, by virtue of his very nature, experiences a central sexual stimulus at the very sight of his own exposed body and so on. Of course, this is considerably increased if masturbation is performed by another suitable individual of one's own sex. In this case, too, the action of the centre is not yet complete. It is only complete to the extent that mutual contact between the two bodies takes place at those points of the periphery which—even in homosexuals—maintain the most direct connection with the centre in sexual feeling, if I may so express myself, that is, namely, the genitals, the mouth (the lips), the inner thighs and palms, then the chest and the front surface of the body in general in contrast to the rear (the back etc.). And because the homosexual differs from the heterosexual only in the one respect expressed by the name but is otherwise equal to him in all relations of sexual feeling—unless his abnormality is accompanied by further exceptional complications, such as fetishism and so on—so also in urning lovemaking the embrace, analogous as far as possible to normal sexual intercourse, is the most natural form of satisfaction. From this it follows that pederasty in the narrow sense [*LATIN: anal penetration*] is actually only significant for normal sexuals who, in the absence of an opportunity for normal satisfaction, are only concerned with a mechanical equivalent for the female genitals, while the body of the male surrogate is otherwise of no interest to them. In the latter case, pederasty is really a kind of unnatural fornication, a designation which even the practitioners of acquired contrary sexual feeling do not deserve, inasmuch as here, too, there is a pathological but nevertheless a physical drive precisely to one's own sex. An original or acquired drive to pederasty, in contrast to a mere occasional utilisation of the anus for the production of a peripheral stimulus, should, however, be counted among the rarities, if one realises that such a drive would require, in addition to the homosexual abnormality in itself, an abnormal behaviour of the—above-mentioned—parts of the periphery, in which sexual sensitivity is embodied in a specific way in homosexuals as well as in heterosexuals.

If these opinions are correct, then this just shows that the German penal legislation relating to unnatural fornication is flawed in the interpretation which, as will be seen from the following quotations, is given to it in the highest judicial instance. For although the homosexual's natural form of sexual satisfaction is the act of coitus, which is analogous to normal copulation, it is precisely this act which is affected by the penal prohibition, while the far more repugnant mutual masturbation, which is also detrimental to health, remains unpunished. Actual pederasty, if only because of its rare occurrence, is of subordinate importance, but in any case, no more unnatural, unhealthy and immoral than other non-punishable indecencies. This is a view which, as can be seen from the following, was already advocated in 1869 by the scientific deputation in Berlin, in the interest of the then imminent new penal legislation, unfortunately without success.

If one examines with impartiality the standpoint which state and society still take in Germany and in some other countries towards being an urning, a knowledgeable person will not be able to avoid admitting that it is rooted in ignorance and blind prejudice. The love of one's own sex is undeniably unnatural in the sense that it runs counter to what we believe to be the plan of nature. But this abnormal direction of the sexual instinct is implanted in the urning by nature itself, and therefore cannot reasonably be regarded as morally reprehensible. Therefore, the Creator, not the creature, deserves to be reproached. It is true that we would always see in Him the loving father. If we—in the more favourable case—are not despised but, as 'unfortunates', pitied, then it is not nature that is to blame for our unhappiness—since we feel at ease in our peculiarity and do not feel the lack of an unknown happiness—but our human judges and persecutors who do not know what they are doing. If the perverted instinct offers opportunity and cause for sexual excesses, it has this in common with the normal sexual instinct. No less than the latter, however, it can be the source of the most blissful happiness as well as of the noblest impulses of the human heart. This view, which has come to the fore in recent scholarship, especially through the author of *Psychopathia Sexualis*, explains the position which being urning occupied even at the time of the flowering of Greece, and which is sufficiently indicated by the one historically transmitted trait from which we learn that Socrates's favourite pupil was allowed to assume that, through bodily devotion to his master, he was rendering him a service of love and himself a merit.

The views that prevail in our state and society are in sharp contradiction with this.

In the 'Motives' to the Prussian penal code, which was valid until 1870 and which punished unnatural fornication with severe punishment, it is stated 'that fornication between persons of the manly (*sic*) sex shows such a great degeneracy and degradation of man and is so dangerous to morality that it cannot remain unpunished'. This view remained untouched until 1870, at least the authoritative one. When the German penal code, now in force, came into force in 1871, the government sought the opinion of the Royal Scientific Deputation for Medicinal Affairs in Berlin on certain matters subject to judicial medical assessment, including unnatural fornication, which had hitherto been frowned upon in Prussia, not without pointing out that such acts were non-punishable in France, Belgium, and even in the legislation of individual German states such as Bavaria. Although the scientific deputation was still far removed from today's scientific standpoint on this subject, the requested expert opinion nevertheless stated that 'this special type of fornication is no different from other, non-punishable acts, whether they are considered to be lewd or unhealthy in their nature'. In particular, if the Royal Supreme Tribunal in various decisions does not accept masturbation practised by men on each other as unnatural fornication between persons of the male sex, the Austrian draft penal law (which deletes unnatural fornication from the number of punishable acts) must be approved. From the point of view of health, it is precisely this masturbation alone that can be given weight, while an imitation of coitus performed between persons of the male sex can essentially only become harmful through excesses, just like ordinary coitus. The expert opinion concludes with the following remark:

> A judgement as to whether fornication committed between persons of the male sex constitutes a particular degradation of man or a particular immorality in comparison with other types of fornication, as they are known to be carried out in the most disgusting manner between men and women or mutually between women, hardly belongs to the competence of the experts. Accordingly, we are not in a position to provide any reasons why, while other types of fornication are disregarded by the penal code, fornication with animals or among persons of the male sex should be punishable.

The legislation did not follow the pronouncements of science. It based this behaviour on the fact that, as it says in the motives for § 175 of the Imperial German penal code: 'The legal consciousness of the people regards these acts not merely as vices, but as crimes'. This view prevailed during the deliberations on the draft law or, perhaps more correctly, it remained unchallenged by the indifference of the majority to this matter, which concerned only a vanishing minority, and could not be influenced even by the arguments of outstanding legal scholars who spoke out in the legal press. To quote only one of the latter, Prof. Dr Sontag of Heidelberg, in Goldammer's *Archiv für preussisches Strafrecht* (Prussian penal law), vol. 18, p. 15, after a preliminary remark on the haste and alacrity with which the German penal code was being drafted, stated, among other things, as follows: 'Despite the objection of the scientific deputation for the medical system, § 143 of the Prussian penal code has been reduced only in its penal measure ... passed into the draft, etc.' Above all, it is almost incomprehensible why the scientific deputation for the medical profession was put into action for this crime, if no consideration was to be given to its vote. The reasons given in the motives (p. 150 ff.) for making sodomy a punishable offence also existed before this enquiry, and if they were really to be considered sufficient, as the authors of the draft believe, then there was no need to demand information from medicine. But now, in order to eliminate the reasons of the scientific deputation, the motives merely refer to 'the people's consciousness'. What this so-called popular consciousness, which has so often made the field of jurisprudence uncertain in recent times, is supposed to mean, is aptly stated by Ahrens (in v. Holtzendorff *Enzyklopädie der Rechtswissenschaft* [Legal studies], Leipzig, 1870, p. 30): 'It behaves with the overall consciousness of the people as it does with Rousseau's general will; as this practically dissolves into the will of all and of the individual, so the consciousness of the individual jurists took the place of the overall consciousness of the people, with whom one could certainly say more often: what bites at the consciousness of the people is fundamentally the spirit of the masters themselves, which is only reflected in the consciousness of the people.' It is precisely in the area of crimes against sexual morality that views are often sharply opposed today and both parties, instead of citing legal grounds, tend to invoke popular consciousness. If only one would finally realise how little this 'chameleon' of popular consciousness means in the legal field; if one would consider that the legislator should not always descend to the people, but in individual cases also pull them up to him, and take to heart the words of Lenz (*Entwurf für Zürich* [Draft for Zurich], p. 24), that 'one would have to forego any progress if one waited with a reform until everyone agreed to it'. After the author has then spoken out against the punishability of 'bestiality' in particular, he goes on to say the following about sodomy between persons of the male sex: 'First of all, it must be noticed that, once one wanted to punish, the Prussian restriction to persons of the male sex was upheld in contrast to almost all German laws and to the very understandable doubt of the scientific deputation' (p. 22 of the appendix in question), whether this kind of sodomy, as opposed to others 'such as are carried out in the most disgusting manner between men and women or mutually between women as is known', constituted a special immorality.

Either all these forms are punishable, or they are all non-punishable. In any case, the latter view seems to be the more correct one. If, as Hälschner (*System des preussischen Strafrechts* [Prussian penal law], III, p. 323) says, simple fornication is an immorality that does not interfere at all with the spheres of the legal system, and therefore lacks the character of illegality and thus also any ground for punishability, then sodomy is no less untenable as an independent crime; this is indeed his view. As long as such acts do not assume the quality of illegality, we may not punish them. The same view is held by Geyer (*Kritik des österr. Entwurfs* [Austrian draft], p. 141), John (*Entw.* [Draft], p. 400), Dalke (*Archiv*, ibid., p. 89). Grolmann, Tittmann and others were in favour of impunity even in earlier times. In addition, such acts are committed among adults by mutual consent and can only rarely be punished, and when they are, they are often based on the most shameful motives. So much for the legal theorists.

According to the interpretation given by the highest German court, the Imperial Court in Leipzig, to the relevant paragraph of the German Criminal Code, unnatural fornication consists of 'acts similar to coitus between persons of the male sex' without restriction to pederasty, including the rubbing or touching of the male member on or with the body of another male person. See *Entscheidungen des Reichsgerichts in Strafsachen* (Decisions of the Imperial Court in criminal matters), edited by members of the Court, Vol. I, p. 395 (*Urt. V. 23 April 1880* [Decision of …]), Vol. II, p. 238 (*Urt. V. 20 September 1880*), Vol. VI, p. 211 (*Urt. V. 25 April 1882*); according to two decisions of the Imperial Court (*Entscheidungen* [Decisions], Vol. XX, p. 225; *Urt. V. 3 February 1890* and *Rechtsprechung des Reichsgerichts* [Ruling of the Imperial Court], Vol. X, p. 416, *Urt. V. 28. May 1888*), the person who inserts the penis of a sleeping person into his own mouth is also guilty of unnatural fornication (incidentally, a decision in which disgust at the repulsiveness of the act seems to have triumphed over internal consistency and which gives rise to suspicions, how great a service would be rendered to the judiciary if, by eradicating § 175 from the penal code, it were to be subjected to the embarrassing duty of sullying its acumen by investigating such abominations, which may present the most diverse variants and thus perhaps just as many problems for legal assessment).

Accordingly, in the present state of jurisprudence, it is no longer correct when it is said in *Psychopathia Sexualis*, 5th edition, p. 274, that [*LATIN: insertion of the penis into a living body*] is part of the offence provided for in § 175 of the German Criminal Code, that the legislator was thinking exclusively of pederasty ([*LATIN: anal penetration*]) and that the criminal punishment of other lewd acts between male persons (insofar as they do not appear to be complicated by a violation of public modesty, the use of force or the performance of such acts on boys under 14 years of age) is therefore no longer applicable.

In fact, it is hard to imagine a more absurd and inherently contradictory legal state than the existing one—even if one disregards the more correct insight into the nature of the contrary sexual feeling, which was only gained after its creation, and which could not yet be granted to the expert opinion of the scientific deputation. It is incomprehensible why unnatural fornication between men should be punishable when that between persons of the female sex is permitted. Although the unnatural lewdness frowned upon by the law is no more immoral than some others, it punishes that and leaves others unpunished. It punishes acts indifferent to health (the imitation of coitus) and permits acts contrary to health (mutual masturbation), which, moreover, are obviously more shameless! If, however, the principle of the punishability of acts similar to coitus is to be assumed, then it is, one may well say, inconsistent to regard the [*LATIN: oral sex*] with a sleeping person as a punishable act—as an analogue of coitus.

In the educated and uneducated public, the idea prevails that love of one's own sex is the product of physical and moral degeneracy and depravity. State and society reinforce each other's prejudices. The legislator invokes 'popular consciousness' and society sees its point of view sanctioned by law and justice and ignores Goethe's parable of the perpetual eternal disease. The judge is the third in this alliance. Anyone who pays attention to the trials of perverse crimes and offences against morality, insofar as they are published, cannot fail to notice that acquittals due to psychopathic conditions of the accused occur in the rarest of cases, but that the consultation of medical experts is also regularly omitted. On the other hand, he will find that severe punishments are usually imposed and that, especially in the case of charges of unnatural fornication, the lowest legal limit of punishment, which consists of one day's imprisonment, does not seem to exist for the judge and is always far exceeded. Unfamiliar with the fact, which has only recently been proved by medical science, that such offences regularly find their explanation in a natural instinct which often even acts with particular strength, the judge follows in good faith the traditional explanation, with which he is exclusively familiar, of the moral depravity of every sexual perversity, and since he does not feel in himself the slightest temptation to violate the moral law on this point, he believes its origin to be in an incalculable abyss of moral baseness, and accordingly reacts against the phenomena rising before him from this dark and uncanny depth, both instinctively and out of conviction, with the whole severity of the means of punishment at his command, comparable to that pious little peasant who, filled with blind faith, brought his piece of wood to the funeral pyre of Johann Huss.[3]

If one considers the overall picture of these views and their consequences from the level of scientific knowledge reached in *Psychopathia Sexualis*, one cannot refrain from seeing a phenomenon of cultural history, remarkable in any case, in a prejudice dominating our enlightened age, which can hardly be reconciled with the facts less than the belief in witches of past centuries and which, like the latter, imposes the harshest trials and persecutions on a blameless minority. This phenomenon can be explained above all by the ignorance of the physiological and psychological facts which morally rehabilitate the urning in the eyes of the expert, and also by the natural aversion which the abnormal instils in the normal sexuals and the tendency to judge one's fellow man, which finds nourishment in the Pharisaic satisfaction of not being like them, finally, by the fact that homosexuals are an overwhelming minority, which is made almost insignificant by the criminal punishment and the general contempt which threatens their members and drives them into secrecy, and which is all the more vividly abhorred by their isolated occurrence.

And now I ask in conclusion: shall this state of things continue? Will not the men who see through the delusion take a hand in destroying it? It is true that those on whom it weighs are unable to do so. They are in a more desperate position than anyone else who is wronged, for they must renounce the defence and the attempt to enlighten their fellow men about the injustice of which they are the authors; by their appearance they would expose themselves to contempt before and without their defence being appreciated. But the men of science cannot and will not shirk this duty assigned to them both by their profession and by the dictates of humanity. The witch mania also seriously gave way to their work. The battle with the prejudice that exists today would be a far easier one, for it is already beginning to be clarified (e.g., the article 'Pederasty' in the latest edition of Meyer's *Großes Konversationslexikon* should be highlighted as a signal of a change in public opinion that is also preparing to take place in wider circles). One would hardly be wrong in assuming that the decision on the incorporation of § 175 into the penal code would have turned out differently today than 20 years ago. Other older and newer penal codes have not included similar provisions and in this respect have a lead over Germany in intelligence and humanity. But if it were easier, the fight for it would be no less meritorious, for the internal and external distress that this prejudice brings upon many innocent people, the victims it drives to despair and death, is no less than the harm once caused by the old delusion, which is incomprehensible to us today. If one considers incidents such as the criminal case of 1888, which is reported in *Psychopathia sexualis*, 5th edition, p. 283, where the authorities intervened against two men because of a tender but completely innocent friendly relationship, put them on trial and sentenced them to a disgraceful punishment, and all this partly on the basis of an 'anal finding', which was a decisive corpus delicti, one will have to admit that between the witch trials of past days and our criminal trials arising from § 175 of the German penal code, there is a not-too-distant similarity, a similarity which even extends to the imaginary evidence on which the 'guilt' or 'innocence' of the 'inculpate' was made dependent. What reasons, then, could prevent men of science from taking serious action against the disaster of which they are eyewitnesses? A book such as *Psychopathia Sexualis* is dedicated to research and is therefore not a suitable subject for popular reading, any more than a work dealing with all the obscene details of normal sexual intercourse would be. But what is to prevent a scholar endowed with the highest authority in his subject from stepping before the public in a discreet manner, with the elimination of adverse details, and instructing them about it: that love of one's own sex is implanted in some of our fellow men by nature, that a natural instinct is no vice or crime, that there are noble, respectable men in whom it is inherent; that it resembles its normal sister as the giver of the highest earthly happiness and as the mainspring of generous devotion to one's neighbour; that society is gravely sinning by the delusion to which it has since sacrificed thousands of blameless brothers and daily sacrifices more every day. The doctor, above all, should devote himself to this task. Not much is lost, even if his art succeeds in individual cases in remedying the perverse impulse; all remedies are at least precarious in the face of the innate impulse, the hypnotic method not excepted—one only has to consider the hardly inferior experiment of imbuing a normal sexual with a contrary sexual feeling through hypnosis. If, however, the doctor were to take it upon himself to free the world from this delusion, he would at the same time be carrying out a mass cure on the deluded and their victims, which would earn him the gratitude of thousands of sufferers. Sooner or later truth and justice will come into play, but I ask again: why does the petitioned doctor hesitate even for a moment to lay hands on the work? Certainly, the activity of the expert who, with the pit light of science, traces pathos into its most hidden recesses, cannot be appreciated highly enough.

But where it is the ignorance of the masses in which suffering, at least on its subjective side, has its real source, he will not be able to avoid the duty of exchanging that pit light for the widely shining torch of popular enlightenment. He will not lack a therapeutic success which would be equal to a progress on the paths of humanity and culture which can never be praised enough!

Notes

1. Throughout this polemic, Symonds uses Ulrichs' word 'dioning' to describe individuals attracted to the opposite sex—or heterosexuals, a word that Krafft-Ebing was already starting to use.
2. The last part of this letter was republished in Richard von Krafft-Ebing, 'Zur conträren Sexualempfindung. Autobiographie und strafrechtliche Betrachtungen von einem conträr Sexualen', *Wiener medizinische Blätter* 15 (1892): 42–44.
3. Jan Huss (1372–1415) was a Bohemian theologian and early church reformer burned at the stake.

CHAPTER 5

For the Good of Science

5.1 PS1 (1886) Bb 23, 64–8

R: *PS2 (1887) Bb 25, PS3 (1888) Bb 31, PS4 (1889) Bb 56, PS5 (1890) Bb 67, PS6 (1891) Bb 80, PS7 (1892) Bb 112, PS8 (1893) Bb 112, PS9 (1894) Bb 109*

I am now 40 years of age, from a perfectly healthy family, have always been healthy, was considered a model of physical and mental freshness and energy, am of strong build, but have only a moderate beard, am hairless on the trunk, except under the armpits and on the pubic area. My penis was already unusually large after birth and is 24 cm long when erect, with a circumference of 11 cm. I am an able horseman, gymnast and swimmer and have participated in two large campaigns as a military doctor. I have never had any taste for female clothing and occupation. Until puberty I was shy towards the female sex and still am towards new acquaintances. I have always had an aversion to dancing.

At the age of eight, my inclination towards my own sex awoke. At first, I enjoyed looking at my brother's genitals. I made my younger brother play with our genitals, which gave me erections. Later, when bathing with the schoolboys, the boys interested me vividly, the girls not at all. I had so little sense for them that even at the age of 15 I believed they also had a penis. In a circle of like-minded boys, we amused ourselves by playing with

D. Pretsell, *Queer Voices in the Works of Richard von Krafft-Ebing, 1883–1901*, Genders and Sexualities in History,
https://doi.org/10.1007/978-3-031-17331-8_5

each other's genitals. When I was 11, I was given a strict school master and could now only rarely steal away to my dear friends. I learned very easily but did not get along with the teacher and when he was too hard on me one day, I went into a rage, stabbed him with a knife and would have stabbed him with lust if he had not fallen into my arm. When I was 12-and-a-half, I ran away from the teacher on a similar occasion and spent six weeks in a neighbouring country.

I now entered grammar school, was already sexually developed at that time and amused myself by bathing with my friends in the manner indicated above, later also by anal intercourse. I was 13 years old at the time. I did not like girls at all. Violent erections caused me to play with my genitals, and I also tried to put my penis in my mouth, which I managed to do by bending over. This caused ejaculations, which led me to masturbation. I was shocked by this, thought I was a criminal and revealed myself to a 16-year-old schoolmate. He enlightened me, calmed me down and made a love covenant with me. We were blissfully happy, satisfying ourselves through mutual onanism. I masturbated at the same time. After two years this covenant was severed, but even today when we meet occasionally—my friend is a senior civil servant—the old fire flares up again. That time with friend H. was a blessed one, whose return I would like to buy with my heart's blood. Life was a joy to me then, learning was fun, and I was enthusiastic about everything beautiful.

During this time, a doctor who was a friend of my father's seduced me by gently caressing me during occasional visits, by masturbating, explaining the sexual processes to me, and admonishing me never to masturbate, as this was harmful to my health. He then engaged in mutual onanism with me, explaining that this was the only way for him to function sexually. He was disgusted by women, which is why he had also lived in discord with his deceased wife. He urgently invited me to visit him as often as possible. The doctor was a handsome man, father of two sons aged 14 and 15, with whom I had a love affair in the following year similar to the one I had had with friend H.

I was ashamed of my infidelity to him, but nevertheless continued the relationship with the doctor. He engaged in mutual masturbation with me, showed me our spermatozoa under the microscope, showed me pornographic works and pictures, which I did not like because I was only interested in male bodies. On the occasion of later visits, he asked me to do him a favour, one he had never enjoyed and for which he lusted. Since I loved him, I conceded everything. He expanded my anus with instruments, then sodomised me while at the same time he masturbated me, so that I felt pain and lust at the same time. After this discovery, I immediately went to friend H., thinking that this beloved man would come to give me even greater pleasure. We sodomised each other, but we were both disappointed and didn't repeat it, because passively I felt only pain and actively no pleasure, while mutual masturbation gave us the greatest pleasure. Only with the doctor, out of gratitude, was I more often at his beck and call. Until the age of 15, I had passive or mutual masturbation with my friends. I was now already an adult, received all kinds of offers from women and girls, but fled them like Joseph fled Potiphar's wife.[1] At the age of 15 I moved to the capital. I only rarely had the opportunity to satisfy my sexual inclinations. Instead, I revelled in the sight of pictures and statues of male bodies and could not refrain from kissing beloved statues. My main annoyance was the fig leaves on their genitals.

At the age of 17, I went to university. For two years I lived with my friend H. again.

When I was 17-and-a-half years of age, I was coerced into coitus with a woman while drunk. I forced myself to do it but was immediately after the act seized with disgust. I fled the house. After this first active attempt at coitus, I felt as if I had committed a crime. In another attempt, made in a sober state, I did not achieve an erection despite all the efforts of the beautiful naked girl, while the mere sight of a boy or the touch of a thigh by a man's hand made my penis stiff as steel. Friend H had recently experienced the same thing. We racked our brains in vain as to the cause. I now let the women be women, found pleasure with friends in passive and mutual masturbation, among others with the two sons of the doctor who had abused them sodomitically after my departure!

At the age of 19 I made the acquaintance of two real urnings.

A., 56 years of age, feminine-looking, beardless, not distinguished mentally, with a strong, abnormally premature sex drive, had been indulging in urning love since the age of six. He came to the capital once a month. I had to sleep with him. He was insatiable in mutual masturbation, also forced me into active and passive sodomy, which I reluctantly accepted.

B., a merchant of 36 years, of thoroughly masculine appearance, was enormously needy, just like I was. He knew how to lend such charm to his manipulation of me that I had to serve him as a catamite. He was the only one with whom I felt some pleasure passively. He confessed to me that just knowing I was near gave him the most embarrassing erection, and if I could not serve him, he had to satisfy himself by masturbation.

Besides these love affairs, I was a clinical assistant in the hospital and was considered zealous and proficient in my profession. Naturally, I searched all the literature for an explanation of my sexual peculiarity. I found it branded everywhere as an offence worthy of punishment, whereas I could only recognise in it the simple, natural satisfaction of my sexual desire. I was aware that this was innate to me, but feeling at odds with the whole world, often close to madness and suicide, I tried again and again to satisfy my powerful sexual urge with women. The result was always the same—either lack of any erection or, if I succeeded, forcing the act. I felt disgust and horror at the prospect of repetition. As a military doctor, I suffered horribly at the sight and touch of thousands of naked male figures. Fortunately, I made a love covenant with a lieutenant who felt the same way about me and once again had a divine time. Out of love for him, I even decided to practice anal intercourse, which his soul craved for. We loved each other until he lost his life at Sedan. From that time on, I never again took to either active or passive sodomy, even though I had many loves and was a very desirable personality.

At the age of 23 I went to the country as a doctor, was sought after and popular, satisfied myself with boys over the age of 14, threw myself into political life, made enemies with the clergy, was betrayed by one of my lovers, denounced by the clergy and forced to flee. The judicial investigation was favourable. I was able to return but was deeply shaken and used the war that had broken out (1870) to serve with arms in the hope of finding death. However, I returned, much decorated, matured into a man, inwardly calm and only found more pleasure in serious, strenuous professional work. I hoped my immense sexual drive was close to extinction, exhausted by the enormous strain of the campaign.

No sooner had I recovered than the old irrepressible urge began to stir again and led to new unbridled satisfaction. Of course, I often stopped to think about myself, to think about the reprehensible nature of my inclination, not in my eyes, but in the eyes of the world.

I abstained for a year with the utmost exertion of my willpower, then I travelled to the capital to force myself to find a wife. I, who was tormented by erections at the sight of the dirtiest stable boy, could hardly achieve an erection with the most beautiful woman. I travelled home devastated and kept a boy for my personal service and satisfaction.

The loneliness of life as a country doctor, the longing for children drove me to marry. I also wanted to put an end to people's gossip and hoped to finally triumph over my fatal urge.

I knew a girl whose kindness of heart and love for me I was convinced of. With my respect and adoration for my wife, I succeeded in coming to terms with my marital duties to produce four boys. The boyish appearance of my wife had a relieving effect. I called her my Raphael, strained my imagination to simulate boyish images and thus achieve erection. But if my imagination lapsed for only a moment, the erection was over. I was not able to sleep with my wife. In recent years coitus has become more and more difficult for me to achieve, and for the last two years we have refrained from it. My wife knows my state of mind. Her kindness of heart and love for me override this.

My sexual inclination towards my own sex is unchanged, and, unfortunately, all too often it has forced me to be unfaithful to my wife. Even today, the sight of a boy of about 16 brings me into violent sexual excitement with embarrassing erections, so that I occasionally help myself by masturbating the boy while I masturbate myself.

The agony I endure is indescribable. For lack of something better, I let my wife masturbate me; but what the woman's hand succeeds with difficulty after half an hour, the boy's hand succeeds after a few seconds! Thus, I live miserably, a slave to the law and to my duty to my wife! I never had any desire for sodomy (active or passive). If I carried it out or tolerated it, it was only out of gratitude, courtesy.

5.2 PS2 (1887) Bb 29, 80–5

R: *PS3 (1888) Bb 41, PS4 (1889) Bb 60, PS5 (1890) Bb 71, PS6 (1891) Bb 84*

My childhood years were probably just as dreamlike and harmless as those of all other people. I received my first impression of sexual life at school around the age of 13. I progressed quickly because I understood very easily and was therefore one of the youngest in the class. Next to me sat a boy who could have been about 15 or 16 years old. After various preliminaries, one day he pushed my hand into his open trousers and let me feel his genitals, which had already developed into an erection. He was probably aiming for masturbatory purposes, but I didn't understand him and just felt a strange intoxicating sensation when touching him.

From this time on, the development of puberty in my classmates and other young people interested me immensely, while I don't remember even thinking about similar processes in the female sex.

At the same time, I had an intimate friendship with a talented boy of the same age, so that we came to be called the lovebirds. There was no trace of sensuality, but on my part a rapturous intimacy, which rose to the level of poems, and I often had violent fits of jealousy when my friend was friendly with other boys.

I was destined to become a merchant and left the grammar school at the age of 16 to enter the factory business of a relative in a neighbouring town. One of the sons of the house was a few years younger than I. We were soon united by a common inclination for artistic matters, both of us having in mind the purpose of renouncing the merchant's profession, I to continue my studies, he to attend the art academy.

For the time being, these beautiful plans, which were strongly opposed by my parents, came to an end when my young friend was sent to W. for a longer period of time to complete an apprenticeship in a friendly house. We corresponded diligently and I eagerly awaited his return.

In the meantime, chance had it that among the young people with whom I was socialising, a person of about 25 years of age was sometimes to be seen, of whom it was secretly said, with expressions of disgust, that he was practising sodomy. I inquired what this meant and was given the usual information that the man in question satisfied his sexual urges with young people's posteriors. I felt an indescribable disgust for the man and avoided him everywhere, although he was quite friendly and mannerly. At that time, it would never have occurred to me that I could have anything in common with him.

In the meantime, I had grown up into a strong young man. Since I never masturbated and felt no inclination to do so, I sometimes had a nightly emission. At first, I paid no attention to the fact that the object of my dreams was always a male being, and I also attributed the excitement I felt when I bathed with other young men, or otherwise happened to see a naked man, to my being so young and reliably hoped that the complete lack of sensual desire for the female sex would develop in time and displace those other impulses.

But I waited in vain. In the meantime, my boyfriend returned from W. I had become almost 19, he over 17. He joined me in the old intimacy, but I discovered to my horror right from the start that I was not just friends with him, but that I loved him passionately. His closeness made me happy, and when I touched him or he jokingly sat on my lap, I could not resist the temptation to press him against me and kiss him, which brought on strong erections. I became very worried about this condition and finally, on the day of my nineteenth birthday, I decided in desperation to consult a doctor.

I chose a renowned doctor who did not know me and told him in great excitement that I had made the discovery that I was not sexually attracted to women but to men. I also mentioned that I only ever embrace and touch male figures in my dreams, and finally asked him for advice. He was of the opinion that I was giving my imagination too much scope; it was quite impossible for a young person of my age to fall into such an aberration, which might occur in older years, but would then bring great misfortune. He advised me not to think about the matter any further, that 'sexual instinct will show me the right way'. He also encouraged me to visit him again from time to time, but I did not do so, as I had become convinced that he could not help me after all.

A short time later, on a trip to the countryside, I had the opportunity to spend the night with my friend in the same room. I could not resist sitting on the edge of his bed and caressing him. He himself asked me to lie down with him and I complied with his permission in the greatest excitement. The utmost displays of tenderness ensued, concluding with a mutual masturbatory outpouring. I was overjoyed and believed that everything was now settled between us. But when I wanted to repeat the matter a few days later, I found less concession and soon my friend explained to me that we had to limit our feelings, men were not allowed to make love to each other, we had to keep our friendship pure from excesses and the like.

I was miserable as hell about it, at any rate just like a lover who had his girl snatched away from him. I had no peace, day and night, suffered from severe chest pains and found relief only in proximity to my friend. He might have suspected something of my state of mind, was friendly and good to me, but as often as I came to him with affection, he refused, not abruptly, but decidedly. He often assured me of his true and sincere friendship and begged me to conquer my passion so that we would not have to part.

My unhappy mood contributed in no small way to my finally devoting myself to my studies. I went to the university, where I enrolled after a short preparation. Half a year later, my boyfriend joined me at university. He had fallen in love with a girl who was not pleasing to his parents, and they removed him to give him other things to think about. By chance, a room was available next to mine and he moved in. Apparently, he was of the opinion that my passion had long since been extinguished. At first everything went well, because I was happy to have him close by and didn't want to anger him or drive him away. But I had my attacks again and pestered him with tenderness and insolence, until he finally preferred to take up other quarters, but without getting angry with me. The separation from my friend had put me in a gloomy mood again, and I had the feeling that I had to do something for myself in this direction in order not to lose all desire for life and striving.

At that time, I still believed that sodomy was something quite different to the feeling that dominated me. I had always been told with certainty that pederasts sought sexual satisfaction in the male anus, whereas this was completely inconceivable to me and the male anus interested me just as little as the female genitalia. I was attracted by the overall appearance of the men I liked. I longed to be near them, to embrace them, kiss them and finally lie with them. If I was allowed to do this, I felt a blissful sensation of touching the body; erection had long since set in and the moment of supreme lust came when only a little friction was needed to bring about the final degree of excitement and effusion. Penetration of the body has never been my wish, although feeling the curves of the backside always gave me a lustful feeling.

At that time, an actor was engaged there who came to be much celebrated. It was not only whispered but openly stated that he was a pederast. After I had tried in vain to meet the gentleman in question somewhere in society, I made the bold decision to go and see him directly. I had visited him twice, under the pretext of hearing his opinion of a friend's work, but I was so inexperienced and shy that I did not know how to make myself understood. Finally, I wrote him a letter in which I bluntly made my real intention known. I really wanted nothing more than a discussion, clarification or relief of my depressed mind, since it had come to me in the meantime that I had to count myself among this detested, despised breed of people. I wanted to see how others came to terms with their lot, and since I had been in the opponents' camp until then, I now wanted to hear the party itself.

This time the actor received me with particular friendliness, he led me into another room than before and introduced me to three or four gentlemen, of whom he told me that they were comrades in fate. My shyness and inexperience, which they did not quite want to believe in, were then ridiculed, but on the whole the conversation remained quite within the bounds of decency. It was towards evening, and some of the gentlemen were getting ready to leave. They asked me to follow them to get to know something of their world. We went into a large public bar where they were joined by several other older and younger gentlemen, some with and some without their darlings, including several non-commissioned officers. I found myself in a magical realm. How unhappy I had felt during this whole time. I had hardly known youthful cheerfulness! And here everything was cheerfulness, exuberance and carefree enjoyment of life. Friendly eyes looked at me with understanding, and that very evening I made the acquaintance of someone who made me forget, at least for a while, all the heartache I had endured.

From time to time I visited the actor who came to be idolised by the ladies because of his beautiful figure. He once said to me: 'You will have a difficult life because you are too much a man of the soul. Your heart is always affected by your love affairs. In our case, that is a double misfortune.'

He was very right.

My profession then took me to another city. After some time, I met a very beautiful and talented musician in the new place, who was unhappy about the fact that he lacked the means to show his talent to its best advantage. I took care of him and, since it could be arranged, I took him into my flat. Things went on for years without a hitch, and he often told me that living with me kept him from dangerous excesses with public girls.

Quite unexpectedly, after a long time, a letter fell into my hands from which it emerged that my friend had been engaged for many months and visited his fiancé every day. He had known how to hide this from me. My mind told me that I must always expect something like this, but the secrecy of the matter and the thought that I had only been the means to an end hurt me unspeakably; there were violent scenes, and I insisted on separation, but he explained to me that he could not yet stand on his own feet, he would not accept good deeds from me if I did not keep him with me; so there would be nothing left for him but to shoot himself through the head. What was to be done? As agonising as the circumstances were for me, I had to stay with him.

The result was that I was seized by a kind of despair. The old struggle was renewed. I travelled to a neighbouring town, went to a doctor, opened myself to him and also insisted on a physical examination. He found everything normal and could only advise me to distract my imagination. I wanted to do this thoroughly. I had already repeatedly tried to let myself be stimulated by women, and now I was looking for a lover to let myself be cured by her. I found a very pretty, good-natured girl who had already had an affair with an officer and now wanted to train for the theatre. Even at the first meeting, I noticed that my lack of interest alienated her, and I thought it necessary to give her a reason for that. Since then, I have been indifferent to all women in a certain respect; but I, myself, wished to put an end to this state of affairs. The guileless creature believed me and was truly devoted to me.

I must expressly say here that women are by no means unsympathetic or even repugnant to me; in the present case, it even gave me a pleasant feeling of comfort to know that I was loved by the simple girl. Her desire to devote herself to the theatre gave me cause for many an instruction, and I tolerated and gladly returned her caresses, but without ever feeling any sexual excitement. In between, from time to time, the indomitable passion for my friend took hold of me. Finally, I decided to use a stronger means. I went on a short trip with the young girl, let on that she was my wife, and lived with her so that I could spend whole nights with her. But all this did not help, and I finally had to realise that my nature would not allow itself to be forced.

Since then, I have no longer bothered myself with such attempts however deeply I lament the fact that the happiness of family life is closed to me. There are young people everywhere who can be persuaded to do us favours.

Fate has given me the opportunity to get to know a very large number of people, and I have always found them to be of the same temperament, with only slight variations. Apart from a few strong distortions, which also occur among female friends, the innermost nature everywhere shows a common tendency towards men.

I have never had any inclination or skill for female handicrafts, nor have I felt any desire to dress in a feminine way; but I have often encountered both hobbies among companions of fate, more or less strongly developed, but mostly among the less educated.

I would also like to mention that my mother was very sad for many years; she gave birth to three children before me, all of whom have married; after me came two more children, who died very young.

My inclination is towards handsome, not-too-strong men, from the time of fully developed puberty to older years. I do not know of any strange passions, but my nature is so resolute that men whom I find unagreeable cannot attract me sensually. I am only very rarely attracted to urnings.

5.3 PS2 (1887) Bb 30, 85–91

R: *PS3 (1888) Bb 40*

I. My parentage, my physical and mental condition and my character: My parents are ordinary, average people, my father phlegmatic, good-natured, yet anxious and soft-hearted, his siblings neuropathic, hypertensive, with normal sexuality. My mother is sanguine, easily irritable, proud, otherwise a very understanding and sensible woman. A distant relative on my mother's side—with whom I have not yet been able to come into closer contact—is probably contra-sexual. My siblings are phlegmatic, average people and happily married. As far as my observations go, there has been no inherited mental illness or death by apoplexy.

I, myself, am not particularly strong physically, but mentally I am up to scratch and am regarded as an ambitious man. My temperament is decidedly sanguine and easily irritable. Generally healthy and feeling at ease, I see as a sign of neurasthenia (whether congenital or as a result of my mental illness to be mentioned later?) the complete paling and trembling in anger, blushing and trembling at great joy, as well as unpleasant heartbeats at encounters with lovers or generally with youths who charm me. For the rest, I am very quick at everything, and, accordingly, expressions that have been used concerning my logic, are 'sensible', 'consistent', 'bold' and 'daring'.

Otherwise, there is nothing conspicuous about me. My clothes are of a masculine cut, my beard is normal, and so on. As a child of six to eight years, I often hung around with girls and was interested in playing with dolls, but the girls were my only companions at that time. However, I never showed any desire or love for crocheting, embroidery or knitting, and did not understand them at all. After the age of seven, I also avoided girls almost as much as other children, and playing soldier was my favourite entertainment for a long time. I always belonged to the highest ranks, but even then, I decided on the promotion of my subordinates, as I now realise, according to the appearance of their faces. In this respect, I am no different from my fated colleagues.

On the other hand, I would like to emphasise the following points as being peculiar to me alone or preferable: as a boy, I took great pleasure in all stages of so-called playing school as well as in such conversations where I had to be a so-called precocious person. I was always the teacher, never the pupil. This was also in keeping with my calm, sedate, precocious nature. Furthermore, it was a peculiarity of mine to have developed too great a consistency in all things (consistent to the point of excess), as well as my own lust for intrigue and the like. At present, I would like to emphasise as a characteristic of mine my reluctance to hunt, to take part in shooting practice, to appear openly before a crowd, to take great pleasure in a race, to take part in riding practice and to appear in a close circle of friends. I may well call myself a sensitive, diplomatic figure, in direct opposition to an openly rakish commander. It should also be mentioned that I do not understand music and painting, while I have a great deal of sense for the practical sciences.

In contrast to the other men, I have never liked dancing, of course with girls and ladies. On the other hand, dancing with young men, especially intellectually awakened youths, would make me feel very at home, and with such youths in tight shirts it would be downright stimulating. It would be most appealing to me if, instead of our frivolous ballerinas, a charming youth were to appear. But this brings me to the second point of my report.

II. My sexual life and feelings: My biography. Since the age of ten, I had repeatedly fallen in love with more or less, but always at least somewhat younger schoolmates, with the onset of violent erections, and in my fourteenth year I had my first intimate relationship with one of them. He returned my love, but in a friendly way, and had no idea of my passion for him, which I didn't even understand at the time. I could kiss and caress him to my heart's content and also received a great many kisses from him. It was the most beautiful time of my life. One afternoon we were lying together in the grass (in the recreation garden of an institution), he on his back, I close to him on his belly, chest to chest, nobody noticed. I embraced his neck intimately and began—I would like to say—to kiss him with all my might. An infinite feeling of delight ran through my body, and instinctively pressing my member against the ground, I lost my innocence. But innocent as my lover was, he did not notice my process; but I did not yet understand it either. Nevertheless, after my innocence was gone, I was overcome by a strange feeling of shame. I ran away and sought a place of decency. For a long time, I no longer kissed my lover, but my passion took over again, and a second time, perhaps even more often, I lay next to him 'in the grass', but already more careful about ejaculating each time. It went on like that for several months. We had to part. The parting was incredibly painful. In the meantime, I also changed my residence, came under different circumstances, learned to forget it—as youth does—and established other relationships.

The latter, however, were of a platonic and ephemeral nature for more than three years. At the age of 18, however, I got to know a young fellow who was hardly 14 years of age, but who was very lovely and well-developed for his age, and with whom I was completely in love within two days. He also liked my 'friendship'. I loved him effusively and without having any qualms about the meaning of this love; all my thoughts were directed towards him, only towards him. My desire was soon enormous and, even if with frequent, longer interruptions, it nevertheless happened very often that in this excitement of mine—as I was taking my cue from a 'grass scene'—I appropriated this and that piece of my idol's clothing, that is, took it to bed with me, in order to wrap myself in it, which was still completely permeated by his fragrant scent, and to caress it—similarly as once 'in the grass'—to quench my desire. Apart from his hat and shoes or even his slippers, every piece of clothing that I had stolen from my beloved in this way seemed to serve me. I didn't think about my actions at all but was rather happy that I could satisfy my desire in this way. The shame I had felt earlier (in my fourteenth year) was also gone, since my beloved could not have known anything about my actions. But I always felt a little distressed at the first encounter after this quenching of desire until I pressed a kiss on his hand or lips again. I had just gone beyond the natural limits of my passion. However, I continued in this way with interruptions for a few years and felt quite well and happy.

But then came a bad time, which I still regret today. I still loved my angel, who in the meantime had only become more beautiful, and could have continued the aforementioned idolatry for a long time (only much later, when I had to learn from his own mouth—terrible to say—that he had often been in the bordello, my love came to an end with infinite pain, but also completely). I was repeatedly teased by my colleagues—especially by one—because of my aloofness towards girls (they knew nothing about my relationship with the aforementioned youth), even ridiculed, and the same colleague called me a 'secret sinner'. But I was not such a sinner, for I loved a beautiful youth so dearly. But I got the unfortunate idea that, since my love did not concern a girl, my action was onanism, and now for more than three years I reproached myself most bitterly and most unhappily, although I had never really masturbated. I suppressed my passion by force. Congestions and pollutions were the result. These, however, came to be taken for a secondary effect of my 'onanism', and soon there was no more disease that I did not imagine. Every pollution that I once managed to suppress from January to April came to be regarded as a step closer to the grave. As fate would have it, I got hold of a booklet on masturbation, written, as I see it today, very darkly and wrongly, and in it I found the greatest reproaches against masturbators, who, because they were not worthy of women, flee them. Leaving my lover, I now sought to love women, but in doing so my condition came to be even more terrible. But I now reproached myself even more, believing that I was no longer worthy of a girl either. And so it went on. I'll stop there, because I still regret this unfortunate time, this unfortunate error and the unfortunate book of an unsuspecting simpleton. Nevertheless, I did not neglect my other duties; indeed, I was all the more eager to get rid of my other thoughts.

By a happy coincidence—and I still praise those days today—I was introduced to Plato's *Symposium* and Jäger's homosexual idiosyncrasy[2] at almost the same time. I was struck by lightning, but an infinitely beneficial lightning, and the scales fell from my eyes. I recovered in the shortest time (everyone was amazed at how well I looked), the mental illness disappeared, and I came to be a man again who respects himself. However, from then on, as seems natural, a certain doggedness and a deep hatred of modern institutions took hold within me.

From then on, I followed my feelings closely and tried to arrange my life accordingly as best I could—unfortunately, it is very difficult. At the same time, I also became an 'actor', that is, in order to mislead my friends and acquaintances, as well as one or the other of the beauties I have my eye on. I seem to speak with great expertise about the beauty of damsels and the like. However, I tend to avoid the girls themselves, not as if I were afraid of them, but because it seems very dishonest to me and is not compatible with my pride to feign love and to behave in a servile manner in front of 'statues'.

To this day, I have not yet succeeded in finding a young man and lover who is like-minded towards me; admittedly, I can rarely get involved in the search for such a one. Nevertheless, I have not given up hope, and this is also the only consolation that keeps me going.

My feeling. In giving a brief description of my feelings, I note first of all that I absolutely do not feel like a woman with regard to the young man—for only to such a man can I show love. This has never been the case. The more charming and calm the young man is, the less warlike and fierce, the better. I always want to lie on his belly, always fall at his feet and lean over him, always worship him, and I would really have to laugh if the young man wanted to reverse one thing or another. This also corresponds to my other characteristics.

Feelings towards the woman. Still slight disgust for the immature, but in any case, plain girl with small breasts, all the more so the high-bosomed maiden, most disgusting the voluptuous woman.

- Aesthetically unattractive (or not suitable for glorification): the breasts, the large pelvis, the sloping shoulders, the feet too small in relation to hips and thighs, the weak bone structure.
- Sensually disgusting (hair-raising): the thought of breasts, the thought of fat calves, in general of all communion with female flesh. Hence my miserable state when I forcibly mingled with the girls and no longer considered myself worthy of them. What a colossal error!

Feelings towards the young man. Even a homely boy, especially one with strong calves. The closer he is to puberty, the more charming. The most attractive is the beardless youth of 16–18 years, some of them almost 'godlike'. The facial features are not secondary, but not decisive. A beautiful mouth, a full hand, a nice foot, a slender build is enough. The fully developed, stocky, bearded man is disgusting. Only once did I like a casual 21-year-old youth with a small moustache and chops. All this, however, is only valid in relation to normal sexual individuals; how it would be with contra-sexuals of different kinds (e.g. man-loving precocious boys, as well as beardless, tender-fleshed men) cannot be stated for lack of acquaintance.

- Aesthetically beautiful (as if made for glorification): the firm chest, the small pelvis, the broader shoulders, the stronger foot, in short, the bone structure that is more proportionate in my eyes.
- Sensually delightful (uplifting and gratifying): the thought of the genitals (especially those untouched by women), the thought of strong calves, in general of the entire, 'virile flesh'. The not yet sexually mature boy is a bud without scent.

Desires, moods and rules of conduct arise from these feelings. First of all, it should be mentioned that I am disgusted by pederasty—as is actually self-evident—but I find contact with a woman even more wicked. In most cases, I would rather undress a beloved young man completely, touch his genitals, lie on him, press myself against him and kiss him intimately. I can safely assume that this would result in ejaculation. I cannot say exactly how often I have such a desire but judging from the pollutions (which usually occur every 8–14 days and thus indicate the upper limit), it is very often. But this only applies as a rule to the majority of the young men! Sometimes, however, that is, in the case of a few particularly decent and graceful young men, it would be an even greater pleasure for me—at least the thought of it is even more delicious—to undress them only from the feet to the genitals and now, lying on my knees in front of them, leaning over them, to embrace their calves and thighs and kiss them from top to bottom in view of their genitals, while the beautiful one would have to exert a slight pressure on my member with the tip of his foot. Why I imagine being on my knees and kissing his calves and thighs to be even more delicious is something I will come to below. But I note again that only very few particularly handsome and honest (naturally untouched) young men seem suitable for such worship, as I may call the process.[3] Finally, it should also be mentioned that young men who hold certain positions, as well as ones in riding costumes, excite me just as much, and the sight of them evokes erections as frivolous girls in tricots do the woman's lover. So to me, breeches and tight-fitting leggings with a short coat seem frivolous, while a decent suit would have to consist of rather wide (about bell-shaped) trousers and a long coat.

If there were a prostitution for youths I would—in the absence of a decent one—make use of it, but in any case, only in the way first indicated. However, I would also know how to treat a decent youth who loves me and could remain faithful to him with ease. In general, I would like to distinguish between equal and not equal, just as normal people do.

After all, it is understandable that, where possible, I spend time in the company of one or the other 'beautiful' person, promenade with him and so on, even though I do not now, and unfortunately have not for a long time, entertained any more intimate 'friendship'. This abandonment often makes me desolate, and only the eternal possibility of hope of better times can bring some reassurance. Apart from that, however, I do not feel unhappy about my love direction, not in the least. Even the thought that I am thereby denied the so-called family joys does not alter me at all. On the contrary, even if I were to imagine that a lover could come to be pregnant (!), I would have no joy at all with him and would not be able to work out how to treat his child, since I do not like to bother with small children up to about two years of age, and especially not with babies. For my part, I would rather devote all my love and care to my beloved in order to train him to be a capable man. If this were to happen, he would have to part with me in any case, but without alienating himself completely from me. He could then take a young man for himself and from one half of the marriage he would become, as it were, the son of my marriage or adopted son; I would then, if I am still young enough, take a second lover, and my greatest pride would be, I already feel, to be able to look down in my old age on a number of capable men who were once my lovers. I would then come to a quiet and contented end of life. But will it come to that?

5.4 PS2 (1887) Bb 37, 98–103

R: *PS3 (1888) Bb 50, PS4 (1889) Bb 44*

Born of healthy parents, I was weak as a child, but thrived under good care and did well at school. In my eleventh year, I was enticed by a playmate to masturbate and surrendered to it with passion. Until my fifteenth year, learning was easy for me. With increasing pollutions, I came to be less proficient, did not do well in school, and was insecure, anxious and embarrassed when called upon by the teacher. Shocked by the permanent decline in my abilities that I had acquired and realising that the great loss of semen was to blame for this, I now refrained from masturbating, but nevertheless the pollutions increased so that I often ejaculated two to three times in one night. I now desperately consulted doctor after doctor. No one could help me.

As I became weaker and weaker due to the loss of semen, and the urge for sexual satisfaction came on stronger and stronger, I went to brothels. But there I could not satisfy myself, for even though the sight of the naked woman gave me pleasure, neither ejaculation nor erection occurred, and even masturbation on the part of the lady did not bring about erection.

No sooner had I left the brothel than I was again tormented by the urge and had violent erections. I was ashamed of myself in front of the girls and no longer visited such houses. A few years went by like that. My sex life consisted of pollutions. My inclination towards the opposite sex grew colder and colder. At the age of 19, I entered the university. I was more attracted to the theatre. I wanted to become an artist. My parents did not agree. In the capital, I had to go out with colleagues to see girls now and then. I feared such situations because I knew that I would not succeed in coitus and that my impotence could be betrayed to my friends, so I did my best to avoid the danger of being ridiculed and disgraced.

One evening, an elderly gentleman sat next to me in the opera house. He flirted with me. I laughed heartily at the foolish old man and went along with his jokes. Suddenly he grabbed my genitals, which immediately caused an erection. Startled, I asked him what he wanted. He told me that he was in love with me. Since I had heard about hermaphrodites at the clinic, I thought I was looking at one, was curious and wanted to see his genitals. The old man happily agreed and went with me to the privy. When I saw the man's remarkably large erect penis, I was frightened and ran away.

The man waited for me, made strange proposals which I didn't understand and rejected. He did not leave me alone. I learned the secrets of male love, felt how my sensuality was aroused by it, but resisted such shameful passion (as I thought at the time) and remained free of it for the next three years. Repeatedly during this time, I tried coitus with girls again without success. Equally unsuccessful were my efforts to rid myself of my impotence through medical science.

When once again sexual libido plagued me, I remembered the old man's lesson that man-loving men get together on the E. promenade. After a terrible struggle and with a beating heart I went there, made the acquaintance of a blond gentleman and let myself be seduced. The first step was taken. This kind of sexual love was adequate for me. I always preferred to be in the arms of a strong man.

Satisfaction consisted in mutual masturbation. Occasionally a kiss on the penis. I was now 23 years of age. Sitting together with my fellow students on the hospital beds during the lectures excited me so much that I could hardly follow the lecture. In the same year, I made a formal covenant of love with a 34-year-old businessman. We lived like man and wife. X wanted to play the man, and I came to love him more and more. I was at his beck and call, but he had to let me be a man now and then. Over time I got tired of him, was unfaithful to him, and he became jealous. There were terrible scenes, temporary reconciliation and finally a definite break-up. (The merchant later became insane and ended his life by suicide.) I made many acquaintances, loved the most vulgar people. I preferred those who were full-bearded, tall and middle-aged, who were good at playing active roles.

I got proctitis. The professor said it was from all the sitting because of the preparations for the exams. I got a fistula and had to have an operation, but that didn't cure me of my urge to be used passively. I came to be a doctor, went to a provincial town and had to live like a nun. I was inclined to move around in women's society and came to be seen with pleasure there, because they found that I was not as one-sided as most men and was interested in toiletries and such ladies' conversation. However, I felt very unhappy and lonely.

Fortunately, I met a man in this town who felt the same way as I did, a 'sister'. He provided for me for some time. When he had to leave, I went through a period of despair with gloom and even suicidal thoughts.

Since I couldn't stand it in the small town, I went to the big city as a military doctor. There I revived, often making two to three acquaintances in one day. I had never loved boys or young people, only real men. That's how I escaped the claws of the police. The thought of falling into the hands of the police was horrible to me; nevertheless, it could not prevent me from satisfying my urges. After a few months, I fell in love with a 40-year-old officer. I remained faithful to him for a year. We lived like lovers. I came to be the wife and was literally pampered by my lover. One day I was appointed to a small town. We were disconsolate. The last night was a constant kissing and caressing.

In T. I was namelessly unhappy, despite some 'sisters' I found. I could not forget my beloved. In order to satisfy the coarse instinct that urged for satisfaction, I chose soldiers. People did everything for money, but they remained cold, and I took no pleasure with them. I managed to go to the capital again. A new love affair, but a lot of jealousy, because my lover liked to go to sisters' parties and was vain and flirtatious. This ultimately led to a break-up.

I was boundlessly unhappy and glad to get away from the capital by transfer. I now sit in C., lonely and desolate. Two infantrymen have been retained, but with the former unsatisfactory success. When will I come to find true love again! I am of medium height, well developed, and look a little worn out, which is why I help myself with makeup when I want to make conquests. Posture, gestures, voice are masculine. Physically, I feel as youthful as a 20-year-old boy. I love the theatre, the arts in general. My attention on the stage is focused on the actresses, on whom I notice and criticise every movement and every wrinkle.

In gentlemen's company I am shy, self-conscious; in the company of my own kind I am boisterous, witty, can flatter like a cat if I like the man. If I am without love, I fall into a deep melancholy, which, however, immediately gives way to the consolations of the first handsome man. For the rest, I am frivolous, nothing less than ambitious. I am not impressed by my job.

Male occupation is unappealing to me. I prefer to read novels, go to the theatre and so on. I am soft, sensitive, easily moved, easily hurt, nervous. A sudden noise makes my whole body tremble, and I have to pull myself together so that I don't cry out.

5.5 PS3 (1888) Bb 34, 87–91

R: *PS4 (1889) Bb 72, PS5 (1890) Bb 89, PS6 (1891) Bb 95, PS7 (1892) Bb 123, PS8 (1893) Bb 123, PS9 (1894) Bb 112, PS10 (1898) Bb 122*

Imbued with the conviction that the riddle of our existence can only be solved or at least illuminated by men of science who think without prejudice, I describe the course of my life solely with the intention of perhaps contributing something to the elucidation of this cruel error of nature and thus possibly being of use to my fellow fates of a later generation; for urnings will come to exist as long as men are born, just as it is an infallible fact that such have existed in every age. But with the advancement of the scientific education of our epoch, one will not see in me and my equals those worthy of hatred, but those worthy of pity, who never deserve contempt, but rather mostly pity from their happy fellow men. I shall communicate with the greatest possible brevity, as well as the strictest objectivity, and note with regard to my drastic, often even cynical style, that I want to be truthful above all, and therefore will not avoid strongly worded expressions, because these characterise most aptly the subject matter I am discussing.

I am 34-and-a-half years of age, a merchant with a moderate income, a little over medium height, lean, have no strong muscles, a full beard and quite an ordinary looking face, and at first sight I differ in nothing from real men. On the other hand, my gait is feminine, especially when walking quickly, my movements are angular and awkward, lacking any masculine grace. My voice is neither feminine nor shrill, rather of a baritone timbre. This is my outward appearance.

I do not smoke or drink, cannot whistle, ride, do gymnastics, fence or shoot, am not at all interested in horses or dogs and have never held a rifle or a sabre. In my inner feelings and sexual desires, I am completely female. Without any deeper education—I only completed five grammar school classes—I am nevertheless intelligent, enjoy reading well-written, tasteful books, have sound judgement, but am always carried away by the mood of the moment and am easily mistreated or incapacitated by anyone who knows my weaknesses and knows how to exploit them. Always making resolutions, I never find the energy to carry them out, am capricious and nervous in a woman's way, often irritable without any reason, sometimes spiteful and arrogant, unjust, often even insolently hurtful towards people who are not in my favour or whom I resent.

In all my doings I am superficial, often frivolous, know no deeper moral feeling, have little tenderness for parents and brothers and sisters, am not selfish, capable of self-sacrifice on occasion, am always persuaded by someone crying and can be won over to anything by kind, courteous or heartfelt pleading—in the manner of a woman.

Even in my earliest years, I withdrew from the war games, gymnastics or scuffles of my male peers, always hung around with little girls I liked much better than with boys, was shy, embarrassed and often blushed. At the age of 12 to 13, the tight-fitting uniform of a handsome soldier already caused me the strangest trepidation, and while in the next few years my schoolmates were always chatting about girls, probably even beginning little flirtations, I was able to follow a powerfully built man with well-developed plump buttocks for hours on end and become intoxicated by the sight of him.

Without thinking much about these impressions, which were so different from the feelings of my comrades, I began to masturbate, always thinking of heroically built, sturdy figures, until I came to know my true condition from a fated comrade in my seventeenth year. Since then, I have had to do with girls eight to ten times, but in order to provoke an erection I always had to think of a beautiful male individual I knew, and I am firmly convinced that today, even with the help of my imagination, I would not be able to use a girl. Shortly after my discovery, I preferred to associate with older, strong urnings, as at that time I had neither the sense nor the opportunity to deal with real men. Since then, however, my tastes have changed completely, and it is only men, real men, between the ages of 25 and 35, with flexible strong builds, who excite my senses to the utmost and whose charms delight me quite as much as if I were a real woman. The circumstances here are such that over the years I have been able to acquire about a dozen male acquaintances who serve my purposes for a fee of one to two guilders per visit. When I am alone with such a handsome young man in a locked room, it gives me above all the greatest pleasure [*LATIN: if his member is large and thick as can be, to take it in my hands and lay hold of it and to press it, to touch his full buttocks and thighs and to feel his whole body with my hands, and, if he lets me, to cover his mouth, face, and his whole body, indeed even his buttocks with ardent kisses. If the member is big and clean, and its master pleases me, then with ardent desire I can give him oral sex for hours. I don't like it, though, if he ejaculates his semen into my mouth, when the majority of those who are called urnings not only enjoy this, but even sometimes swallow semen.*] I feel the most intense lust, however, when I encounter a real man trained in this way [*LATIN: who receives my member into his mouth and allows an erection in his own mouth.*]

As improbable as it sounds, I always find a few good fellows who are willing to be used for a tryst. They usually get to know the story in the military, because the urnings know that people are most compliant for money there, and once the lad is trained, he is sometimes induced by circumstances to continue the thing, despite his passion for the female sex.

With few exceptions, urnings leave me cold, because anything feminine repulses me to the highest degree. Nevertheless, there are some among them who can enchant me quite as much as a real man and with whom I prefer to consort for the reason that they sometimes return my ardent caresses just as passionately. In a tête-á-tête with such an individual, I do not put any restraints on my excited senses, I allow my animal instincts to run riot. [*LATIN: I kiss, I press, I embrace him, I insert my tongue into his mouth; with a mouth trembling with desire I suck on his upper lip, I apply my face to his buttocks, and if a pleasurable scent emanates from his buttocks, then I am overcome with pleasure*]. Real men in tightly fitting uniforms make the greatest impression on me, and if I have the opportunity to embrace and kiss such a handsome man, I immediately ejaculate, which I attribute to my frequent masturbation. For I used to do this very often in earlier years, almost every time I saw a handsome man I liked, whose image then floated before my eyes while I was masturbating. My taste is by no means simple, like that of a servant girl who dreams of her ideal in a strapping dragoon sergeant. A beautiful face is a pleasant addition, but by no means indispensable to inflame my sensual desire, but the main thing remains: [*LATIN: a man whose lower body is robust and nicely shaped, with bulging thighs and hard buttocks*], while the upper body can be slender. A big belly disgusts me, a sensual mouth with fresh breath excites me in the most tingling way, and if such an individual also has [*LATIN: a beautiful, large, and evenly shaped member*], all my—even the most far-reaching—demands are fully satisfied.

With men who please me and excite me passionately, I used to ejaculate five to eight times during one night, even now four to six times, because I am unusually horny and sensually inclined, and even the clashing of sabres of a dashing hussar can excite me. At the same time, I have a very vivid imagination, think of beautiful men with strong limbs almost in all idle hours and would watch with rapture if a strapping firm fellow bursting with strength [*LATIN: endowed with a large penis, might fuck a girl in my presence. I'm convinced that at this sight my senses would be affected by a most intense passion and that while he fucked, I would touch the beautiful young man's body and, if it should be permitted, that I would climb on top of him as he lies with the girl and that I would do the same thing with him and insert my member into his arse.*] At present, only my limited financial means prevent me from carrying out these cynical plans—of which my thoughts are very often filled—otherwise I would have realised them long ago.

The military exerts the greatest charm on me, but I also have a particular soft spot for butchers, cabbies, firemen, circus riders and ship captains, but they all have to be robust and powerfully built. I hate urnings for intimate friendship, as I have an inexplicable, completely unjustified aversion to most of them. With only one exception, I have never been on intimate terms with an urning. On the other hand, I have had the warmest long-term relationships with a few men of the same age, in whose company I feel very comfortable, but with whom I have never had sexual intercourse and who have no idea of my condition.

Conversations about politics, economics and any discussion of a serious topic are abhorrent to me, but I chatter about theatre with a fair amount of understanding and a significant preference. In operas, I see myself on the stage, feel myself being swept away by the applause of the frenzied audience and would love to sing passive heroines or dramatic female roles.

But the most interesting topic of conversation for me and my fated companions is always our men; this subject is inexhaustible for us and their most secret charms come to us in minute detail. [*LATIN: We estimate the size and thickness of their penises; we compare their shapes and how hard they get; one learns from the other who cums faster, who slower.*] I would also like to mention that of my four brothers, one has allowed himself to be used for urning purposes without being an urning himself, and all four are passionate lovers of women who constantly engage in sexual excesses. The genitals of the men in our family are, without exception, strongly developed.

In conclusion, I repeat the words with which I began these lines. I did not censor my language because I was concerned to provide material for the study of an urning existence, in which absolute truth is of primary importance.

To this circumstance I ask you to excuse the numerous crudities.

The writer of these lines is a character of unquestionable integrity, and if you would like further clarification, or to know the correct name, I would kindly ask you to let me know by writing to X.

5.6 PS4 (1889) Bb 66, 149–51

R: *PS5 (1890) Bb 83*

My recent abnormality consists in the fact that I feel completely female in sexual relations. Since my early youth, I have only ever had images of males and male sexual parts before my eyes in my sensual actions and fantasies. Up to university I found nothing remarkable about this (I had never spoken to others about my fantasies, but rather lived a very closed and withdrawn life at grammar school). At university I noticed that females did not excite me in the least. Since then, I have often tried in brothels and other places to engage in sexual intercourse or even achieve an erection with women, but so far always in vain. Every erection was lost as soon as I was alone in a room with a female. At first, I thought this was impotence, while at the same time I was so sexually aroused that I had to masturbate several times a day to be able to sleep.

My feelings towards the male sex, however, developed in a completely different way, and more strongly with each passing year. In the beginning, they expressed themselves in the feeling of a tremendously enthusiastic friendship for certain personalities under whose window I waited for hours at night, whom I met in the streets in every possible way and with whom I sought to come into contact again and again. I wrote the most passionate letters to such persons, in which, however, I shied away from expressing my feelings too clearly. Later, in my twenties, I came to realise the sensual nature of my inclinations, mainly through the sensation of desire I felt as soon as I came into direct contact with any of these friends. These persons were all beautifully built men, with dark hair and eyes. I never felt stimulated by boys; actual pederasty is completely incomprehensible to me.

Around this same time (22–23 years of age), the circle of people I loved expanded more and more. Now I can hardly look at a handsome man in the street without the desire coming to me to possess him. I love mainly people of the lower classes, whose strong forms attract me: soldiers, guards, tramway drivers and so on, especially anyone who wears uniforms. If one of them returns my gaze, I feel a kind of shiver through my whole body. In the evening in particular, I am aroused, and the powerful footfall of a soldier alone can cause me to get the strongest erections. It is my own kind of pleasure to follow and look at such people. As soon as I learn that they are married or that they have affairs with girls, my excitement usually ceases.

Until a few months ago, I was able to control my inclinations to such an extent that I did not make them directly noticeable. Around this time, however, a soldier I was following seemed inclined to respond to my wishes, and I approached him. For money, he was ready for anything. I was immediately filled with the most intense desire to embrace and kiss him, and I did not let the danger of drawing attention stop me from doing so. He had hardly taken hold of my genitals when I immediately ejaculated. With this encounter I had finally understood the goal of my whole life, which I had felt for a long time. I knew that my whole nature would find happiness and satisfaction in it, and I resolved from then on to strive only to find a person whom I could love and from whom I would never separate again. I do not feel the slightest remorse about my actions.

However, in so-called quiet moments I feel very well the great difference that exists between my way of thinking and the views of the world, and as a lawyer, I also naturally know the dangers of a relationship as I wish, but as long as my whole nature does not change, I will not be able to resist the temptations that confront me. Despite all this, I would be prepared to submit to any cure in order to get out of my abnormal state.

I recognise that I feel feminine, among other things, by the fact that every sensual idea in connection with a lady would appear to me to be almost forced and contrary to nature. I am also sure that my respect for a woman—I spend a lot of time in women's company and feel very comfortable in such company—would immediately turn into reluctance if I were to notice any sensual inclinations towards me from such a woman. In my dreams and sensual fantasies of men, I always think of myself in such positions with their faces turned towards me. My delight would be at its highest if a strong man, undressed, were to press me into his arms with a force I could not resist. In general, I think of myself in a passive role in such situations, and I would have to force my feelings to think of myself in a different position. I am truly feminine and shy in this. As great as my desire may be to approach this or that personality, just as great is my endeavour not to let this inclination be noticed. Moustaches, thick hair, even dirt seem particularly attractive to me. I hardly need to notice that my condition, in the face of social considerations, seems to me to be quite desperate, and if

I did not have the hope of still finding someone who understands me, I would hardly be able to bear life. I feel that sexual intercourse with men is the only means of effectively counteracting my tendency to masturbation. Although I often experience this tendency, I cannot refrain from it in the long run, because otherwise, as I have often experienced, I would only become weakened even more at night by pollutions and during the day by erections that last for hours.

I have only ever truly loved two men. Both were officers, excellently gifted, beautiful and slim, brunette people with dark eyes. I met the first one at university. I was madly in love with him, suffered unspeakably from his indifference and spent half the night under his windows just to be near him. When he departed, I fell into despair. Soon afterwards, I met an officer similar to him, who also captivated me from the first moment. I sought out every opportunity to meet him, spent the whole day on the street and in places where I could hope to come to see him. I felt the blood rush to my face when I saw him unexpectedly. When I saw him socialising with others, I could hardly contain my jealousy. When I sat near him, I wanted to touch him; I could hardly hide my excitement when I touched his knees or thighs. However, I was never able to express my feelings to him, because I had to assume from his behaviour that he would not have understood or shared them. I am 27 years of age, of medium height, well developed, am considered attractive, have a somewhat narrow chest, small hands and feet and a weak voice. I believe that I am intellectually well-disposed, since I passed the state examination with distinction, speak several languages and am a good musician.

In my profession, I am considered to be hard-working and conscientious. My acquaintances find me cold and strange. I don't smoke, don't do any sport, can't sing and can't whistle. My gait is somewhat stilted, as is my speech. I have a great sense of elegance, love jewellery, sweets and perfumes, and like to socialise with ladies.

5.7 NF (1890) Bb 2, 43–6

R: ***NF (1891) Bb 3***

Considering that my mother tongue is Hungarian, please excuse my German spelling, which may not always be correct.

I am a civil servant with a small income, and I am currently 39 years of age. Probably the most remarkable thing in my life story is the certainly rare circumstance that I reached the age of 34 without knowing myself and my nature. I do remember from my youth that sexual intercourse with girls never gave me the pleasure that my peers and friends spoke of with so much delight. I also know for certain that from my earliest youth, my dreams only showed me men, but despite all this I remained completely unenlightened.

From my earliest youth I was a dreamer and inclined to melancholy. I was also well aware that something was not right with me, but I was dominated by the belief that I was probably the only one who, in my opinion at the time, felt so unnatural, and for that reason I was careful not to reveal anything about my strange feelings to even my most intimate friends.

Like my peers, I went with girls from time to time and had intercourse with them without horror, but also without blissful pleasure. I also had serious love affairs with various girls and women, in which—as I now explain the matter to myself—friendship on my part and love on theirs were probably combined. One girl, whose true love I did not reciprocate, ended in suicide because of it. A 30-year-old woman, with whom I had a shameful relationship in my twenty-seventh year, divorced her husband out of love for me and subsequently embittered my life for a long time, because I refused to marry her. Two years later I made the acquaintance of a girl I liked and decided to marry her.

I loved my wife truly and sincerely in the beginning, fulfilled my husbandly duty faithfully and would probably have remained unenlightened or undiscovered until the end of my life if my marriage had been happy; but it was not. My wife suffered from hysteria and tormented me so terribly for no reason at all that our marriage, which incidentally remained childless, dissolved after three years. It ended in divorce at my request, against my wife's will.

Around that time, a royal scandal took place in B., and the more or less spicy glossy reports that appeared in the newspapers at that time first opened my eyes a little. More and more I felt the irresistible desire to hold a young man close to me and kiss him, but where to find him? As fate would have it, I was travelling through Vienna when, late one evening, at a urinal, I noticed the demanding eyes of a man I quite liked. That moment decided the rest of my life.

A few minutes later we were acquainted; but what I felt then cannot be described by my feeble pen. It was as if I had awakened after a long sleep. Of course, he didn't believe that I was doing it for the first time in my life and told me quite openly that it was a dull way of making things interesting. But I was enlightened and knew that I was not alone, and I had only one thought—to get to know the mysteries of my sex that had remained closed to me until then.

Partly by chance, partly by clumsiness, I was initially only able to find subjects whose social position and education were far below mine. I became disgusted with myself, despised myself and thought of suicide. All efforts to turn back were in vain; I could no longer bring myself to have intercourse with women and felt immensely depressed in the consciousness of an imagined moral defect.

But this lasted only until fate brought me a truly intelligent and sincere friend who completely cleared up my ignorance, gave me relevant books to read and initiated me into all the necessary secrets. I joined him in intimate friendship and still enjoy it today, although the desire for mutual possession ceased after only a few weeks. I now found myself in a new world; I heard of so many who all felt as we both did and were happy and full of life. The thoughts of suicide gave way, and I abandoned myself to the pleasures that had remained unknown to me until then.

It was not long before I was more or less acquainted with, and befriended, all the people of my father's town. Four years have passed since then; I could no longer say with how many I have enjoyed the highest bliss since then; only it seems quite unbelievable to me today that I had lived so long unenlightened, as if in a dream. I could no longer have intercourse with women, nor have I even attempted it.

If I were not constantly tormented by the fear of being discovered, I would feel, if not happy, at least better than before. Partly my past life, partly my caution will probably keep me from being discovered in the future.

I am attracted exclusively to young, nicely dressed people with moustaches. I am completely indifferent to people who have a full beard or who have already passed the age of 30; I don't notice them at all.

For a year now, a young friend has been making me happy, without possessing this nature himself, merely out of friendliness, arising from various services rendered to him by me. I love him platonically, that is to say, I touch and kiss him, whereby I ejaculate without his having any idea of it.

With other young people, called 'intelligent'[4] by us, I satisfy myself by imitating coitus between the legs. Pederasty arouses a feeling of disgust in me. I am amazed that despite my 39 years and my rather aged appearance, I still find enough young companions of fate who strive to please me quite unselfishly. The fact that my outer appearance does not reveal my inner self in the slightest may contribute a great deal to this, and that this is a quality that is as rarely encountered as it is generally desired. I possess only one female characteristic, about which, however, no one knows anything, namely, I have a special predilection for cooking and would certainly have gone far as a cook.

As far as the observations I have made so far concerning my fated friends are concerned, I have to say that most of them are awfully superficial people who are only good for gossip and not for serious conversation. Most of them never come to realise their condition, have never read a word about such things, but are almost without exception good-hearted and of an exceedingly soft disposition. This is the rule, but there are exceptions. There are also people who are absolutely intellectually gifted. I now know most of Vienna, Budapest and Graz and can say that there is probably no profession or trade in which we are not represented.

If I knew that my condition could be cured by suggestion, I would gladly submit to any torture.

I am healthy, by the way, and know nothing of any illness, except that for two years I have not tolerated the slightest pressure on the region of my stomach, which is why my trousers and coat must always be kept as loose as possible. If, for example, I were to tie my pants even so lightly, I would get fainting fits, especially after eating. Perhaps this is also a neurasthenic condition, but it is not unbearable.

Finally, I would like to mention that I did not masturbate either in the unenlightened or later in the enlightened state, and that my relative well-being can perhaps be traced back to this condition.

I believe you will come to the conclusion from my biography that, if in anyone, then certainly in me, the condition is innate. Unfortunately, I don't know anything about my parents or grandparents; I was completely orphaned at the age of four. I only learned that my mother was my father's third wife, and in this late marriage I was the fifth and last child. Shouldn't the idea suggest itself that such cases are perhaps most likely to arise where the procreative power of the man is significantly inferior to the procreative power of the woman? I know of two other cases where this is really true, namely, where the father was much too old and worn out compared to the mother. But then the child would have too much of the mother and too little of the father.

Notes

1. This is a biblical reference. Potiphar's wife attempted to seduce Joseph, and when he resisted, she accused him of rape resulting in his imprisonment (Genesis 39: 5–20).
2. This is the first use of the word 'homosexual' in Krafft-Ebing's works. The author is referencing Gustav Jäger's *Die Entdeckung der Seele*, which included a section on the homosexual written by Karl Maria Kertbeny.
3. It should be mentioned that I am not interested in reciprocal manustupration (so-called mutual masturbation). I would rather imitate the position and movement of a man during coitus.
4. The word used here is 'vernünftig'. According to Ulrichs, this word was used as a euphemism for urning/homosexual. Karl Heinrich Ulrichs, *Memnon, Abtheilung II*. Schleiz: C. Hübscher'sche Buchhandlung, 1868. Translated by Michael Lombardi-Nash as 'Book Seven: Memnon II' in *The Riddle of 'Man-Manly' Love: The Pioneering Work on Male Homosexuality*, vol. 2 (Buffalo: Prometheus Books, 1994), 494n21; Letter 151 in Douglas Pretsell, *The Correspondence of Karl Heinrich Ulrichs, Karl Heinrich, 1846–1894* (Cham: Palgrave Macmillan, 2020), 195.

CHAPTER 6

The Women

6.1 PS4 (1889) Bb 42, 76–7

R: *PS5 (1890) Bb 51, PS7 (1892) Bb 95, PS8 (1893) Bb 95, PS9 (1894) Bb 95, PS10 (1898) Bb 105*

[KRAFFT-EBING: Ilma S., 29 years of age, single, daughter of a merchant, comes from a heavily encumbered family. Father was a drinker and ended by suicide, as did the patient's brother and sister. Sister suffered from hysteria convulsiva. Mother's father shot himself in a state of insanity. Mother was sickly and died apoplectically paralysed. Patient was never seriously ill, gifted, enthusiastic, imaginative, dreamy. Menses at 18 years without complaints, subsequently highly irregular. At the age of 14 chlorosis and fright catalepsy. Later hysteria gravis and attacks of hysterical madness. At 18, relationship with a young man, which did not remain platonic. This man's love was returned fervently. From hints given by the patient it is clear that she was very sensual and, after distancing herself from her lover, gave herself up to masturbation. Patient subsequently led a novel lifestyle. In order to get ahead, she put on men's clothing, became a tutor, gave up the job because the woman of the house, not knowing her sex, fell in love with her and stalked her. She then became a railway official. In the company of her colleagues, in order to conceal her true sex, she had to visit brothels with them and listen to the most indecent conversations. This became so disgusting to her that she gave up her

D. Pretsell, *Queer Voices in the Works of Richard von Krafft-Ebing, 1883–1901*, Genders and Sexualities in History,
https://doi.org/10.1007/978-3-031-17331-8_6

job, put on women's clothing again one day and sought her livelihood in a woman's position. She was imprisoned for theft and hospitalised for severe hystero-epileptic insults. She was discovered there to have an inclination and drive towards her own sex. The patient was a nuisance everywhere because of her sexually obvious love for nurses and fellow patients. Her sexual perversion was thought to be congenital. Patient gave interesting corrective explanations in this respect:]

One judges me incorrectly if one believes that I feel like a man towards the female sex. Rather, I behave as a woman in my entire thinking and feeling. After all, I loved my cousin as only a woman can love a man.

The change in my feelings came about because in Pest, disguised as a man, I had the opportunity to observe my cousin. I saw that I had been badly mistaken about him. This caused me terrible anguish. I knew that I would never be able to love a man again, that I belonged to those who love only once. In addition, I had to listen to the most disreputable conversations and visit the most disreputable houses in the company of my colleagues from the railway. The insights I gained into the goings-on of the male world gave me an insurmountable aversion to men. But since I am by nature very passionate and have the need to attach myself to a beloved person and give myself completely to her, I felt more and more powerfully attracted to women and girls I liked, especially those who were distinguished by intelligence.

[KRAFFT-EBING: The apparently acquired contrary sexual sensation of these patients often expressed itself in a stormy, decidedly sensual manner and gained further ground through masturbation, since the permanent supervision in hospitals made sexual satisfaction with one's own sex impossible. Character and mode of occupation remained feminine. There were no manifestations of pronounced masculine qualities.]

6.2 PS4 (1889) Bb 79, 173–4

R: PS5 (1890) Bb 97, PS6 (1891) Bb 103, PS7 (1892) Bb 128, PS8 (1893) Bb 128, PS9 (1894) Bb 124, PS10 (1898) Bb 135, PS11 (1901) Bb 158

[KRAFFT-EBING: C. R., maid, 26 years of age, has been suffering from paranoia originaria and hysteria since her developmental years, had a novelistic past due to her delusions, and in 1884 came under judicial investigation in Switzerland, where she had fled due to delusions of persecution. On this

occasion it was discovered that R. was afflicted with contrary sexual feelings. No information is available about her parents and relatives. Apart from pneumonia at the age of 16, R. claims never to have been seriously ill in the past. First menstruation at 15 without any complaints, subsequently often irregular and abnormally strong. The patient affirmed that she had never felt any inclination towards persons of the opposite sex and had never tolerated the approach of a man. She had never been able to understand how her friends could discuss the beauty and loveliness of male persons. She could not understand how a woman could let herself be kissed by a man. On the other hand, she was delighted and thrilled to press a kiss on the lips of a beloved friend. She had an incomprehensible love for girls. She had loved and kissed some friends with rapture; she could have laid down her life for them. Her greatest wish would have been to live permanently with such a friend, to possess her completely.

She felt like a man towards the beloved girl. Even as a little girl, she had only had a taste for boys' games, loved shooting and military music, had always been enthusiastic about such things and would have liked to have gone along as a soldier. Hunting and war were her ideals. In the theatre, she only had a taste for the female actors. She knew that this whole direction was unfeminine, but she couldn't help it. Walking in male clothing was a great pleasure for her, and she had always preferred to do male work and showed particular skill in it, especially manual labour, while she had to claim the opposite with regard to female work. Patient also loves smoking and alcoholic drinks. Due to persecutory delusions, in order to escape supposed persecutors, patient has repeatedly moved about in men's clothes and male roles. She did this with such (probably innate) skill that she was generally able to deceive people about her true sex.

It has been established in the files that the patient moved around for some time in 1884, sometimes in civilian clothes, sometimes in a lieutenant's uniform, and fled to Switzerland in August 1884 in a man's suit, such as those worn by servants of the ruling class, out of delusions of persecution. There she found a job in a merchant's family and fell in love with the daughter of the house, the 'beautiful Anna', who in turn, not recognising the true sex of R., fell in love with the handsome young man. Patient makes the following characteristic remarks about this episode:]

I was completely in love with Anna. I don't know how this came about and can give myself no account of this inclination. In this fatal love lies the reason that I have continued to play the role of a man for so long. I have never felt love for a man and believe that my love is directed towards the female and not the male sex. I am quite unclear about this state of mine.

[KRAFFT-EBING: R. wrote letters to her friend Amalie from Switzerland, which were enclosed with the court documents. They are letters of a rapturous love that goes far beyond the scope of friendship. She apostrophises her friend:]

My wonderful flower, the sun of my heart, the longing of my soul.

[KRAFFT-EBING: She was her greatest happiness on earth, her heart belonged to her. Letters to her friend's parents also say that she would also like to see her 'miracle flower', because if she were to die, she would no longer be able to bear life.

R. spent some time in an insane asylum to have her mental state examined. When Anna was admitted to visit R., there was no end to the fiery hugging and kissing. The former blatantly admitted that they had already embraced and kissed each other at home with the same tenderness.

R. is a tall, slender, stately figure of a thoroughly feminine build, but with more masculine features. Skull regular, no anatomical signs of degeneration, genitals quite normal and quite virginal. R. gave the impression of a morally uncorrupted and decent personality. All circumstances indicated that she had only loved platonically, her look and appearance pointed to a neuropathic personality. Severe hysteria, at times convulsive seizures with visionary and delirious states. The patient is very easily brought into somnambulism by hypnotic influence and in this state is capable of all possible suggestions. (My own observation. Friedreich's Blätter *1886. Issue 1.)]*

6.3 PS9 (1894) Bb 119, 285–8

R: *PS10 (1898) Bb 129, PS11 (1901) Bb 152*

[KRAFFT-EBING: Miss L. 55 years of age. There is no information about her father's family. Her mother's parents are described as angry, capricious and nervous. One of her mother's brothers was epileptic, another was eccentric and mentally abnormal. Her mother was sexually hyperaesthetic and for a long time Messaline.[1] *She was considered psychopathic and died of brain disease at the age of 69.*

Miss L. developed normally, had to endure only minor childhood illnesses, was mentally very gifted, but of neuropathic constitution, emotive, plagued by all kinds of tics. At the age of 13, still two years before her first menstruation, her first love passion for a girl of her own age awoke 'a dreamy feeling, still completely pure of sensuality'. The second love was for an older girl who was a newlywed, with already tormenting sensual longing, jealousy and the still 'unclear feeling of mysterious impropriety'; rejected by this lady, the patient fell in love with a happily married woman and mother 20 years older. She was able to control her sensual impulses, so that this woman never suspected the true reason for such a rapturous 'friendship' and gladly granted it to her for 12 years. The patient describes this long period as a true martyrdom.

In the last few years, from the age of 25, she had begun to satisfy herself through masturbation. At that time, the patient seriously considered whether marriage could save her, but her conscience spoke against it, for she might have passed on her unhappiness to children or 'made a trusting man unhappy'.

At the age of 27, a girl approached her with undisguised proposals, described the nonsense of renunciation, gave full disclosure of the homosexual urge that dominated her, and was very passionate. The patient tolerated this girl's caresses, but did not allow herself to have sexual intercourse, as she felt that her sensual pleasure was repulsive without a passion for love.

The patient spent years mentally and physically unsatisfied, conscious of a failed life. She fancied ladies of her acquaintance from time to time, but knew how to control herself. She was also able to free herself from masturbation.

At the age of 38, Miss L. met a girl 19 years younger, of rare beauty, but from a demoralised family, seduced by cousins into mutual masturbation at an early age. It is not possible to decide whether this girl, A., was a case of psychic hermaphroditism or one of acquired contrary sexual feeling. The former assumption is the more probable. From an autobiography of L. the following emerges:]

A., my pupil, began to turn her idolatrous love towards me. I liked her very much. Since I knew that she had a hopeless love affair with a wild journeyman and continued to have intimate relations with her demoralised cousins, I did not want to push her away. Pity and the conviction that she was otherwise heading for moral ruin prompted me to tolerate her approach.

I did not consider her inclination towards me dangerous, since I did not think it possible that (in view of their love relationship) two passions (for a man and a woman at the same time) could exist in one soul; moreover, I believed I was sure of my power of resistance. So I kept A. around, renewed my moral resolutions and considered it a duty to use A.'s love for me for her ennoblement. What a foolish delusion this was, I was to learn only too soon. Once, when I was asleep, A. knew how to satisfy her lust for me. If I had awoken in time, and if I had been morally stronger, I could still have rejected her. But I was terribly excited, as if intoxicated—she won.

What I felt afterwards is indescribable. Lamentation over the broken resolution that I had upheld with such great effort until then, fear of discovery and of contempt, jubilation at finally being free of the agonising vigil and struggling, unspeakable sensual pleasure, anger at the unfortunate companion and at the same time the feeling of the deepest tenderness. A. calmly smiled at my emotional agitation and tried to calm me down by caressing me.

I found my way into the new situation. Our companionship lasted for many years. We lived on in mutual masturbation, never excessively or lasciviously.

Gradually the sensual intercourse between us ceased again. A.'s tenderness tired, but mine remained, although I no longer felt any sensual desire. A. made plans to marry, partly to be provided for, but essentially because her sensuality returned to normal. She succeeded in finding a husband. May she make him happy, which I doubt. So I have the prospect of dragging my old age along just as joylessly and restlessly as was the case in my youth.

With melancholy I remember the years I spent together with my beloved. The fact that I had sexual relations with A. does not weigh on my conscience, for I succumbed to her seduction and made a sincere effort to save her from moral ruin and to educate her to become an educated and well-mannered being, which I also succeeded in doing. Moreover, I am reassured by the thought that moral laws can only be devised for normal people, but not binding for abnormal ones. Sensitive people who know they are outcast from nature and abandoned to contempt by culture can never be completely happy, but there was a wistful calm in me, and, at moments when I thought A. was happy, I was temporarily happy.

This is the story of an unhappy woman who, through a fatal freak of nature, is cheated of all joy in life and consigned to grief.

[KRAFFT-EBING: I got to know the writer of this story of life and suffering as a finely educated personality, with coarse features and a strong-boned but thoroughly feminine physique. She has been through menopause for a few years without any particular complaints and has felt free of sensual impulses ever since. She has never felt sexually in a certain role towards her beloved woman; she has never felt any sensual impulse towards men.

When asked about the family and health conditions of her former lover A., Miss L. provided information from which a heavy burden appears without a doubt, insofar as her father died in an insane asylum, her mother was in the menopausal stage and neuroses occurred several times in the family and A. had suffered from severe hysteropathy[2] *with occasional hallucinatory delirium for a long time.]*

6.4 PS10 (1898) Bb 132, 263–4

R: *PS11 (1901) Bb 155*

[KRAFFT EBING: Homosexuality. Miss X., from a bourgeois family in a large city, was 22 years of age at the conclusion of my observation. She is considered a beauty, is idolised by men, is of a decidedly sensual nature, was created as if she were an Aspasia,[3] *but refused all the proposals made to her. Only for one of her admirers, a young scholar, did she show a willingness, became intimate with him, allowed him kisses, but not like a loving woman, and when Mr T. once thought he was close to the goal of his desires, she tearfully begged him not to do such a thing to her, since she was absolutely incapable of it, not for moral reasons, but for deeper spiritual ones. The unsuccessful rendezvous was followed by confidences by letter, which led to the certain conclusion of contrary sexual feelings.*

*Miss X. comes from a father devoted to [*LATIN: drinking*] and a hysteropathic mother. She is of neuropathic constitution, has full breasts, is the outward appearance of a woman of rare beauty, but is conspicuous by her tomboyish nature, has decidedly masculine inclinations, performs gymnastics, rides, smokes, has a strapping appearance and a decidedly masculine gait. She wants to devote herself to the stage. Recently, she has become conspicuous through enthusiastic friendships with young ladies. She has one of these with her and shares a place with her.*

*Until puberty, Miss X. claims to have been completely indifferent sexually. At the age of 17, she made the acquaintance of a young foreigner at a seaside resort, whose 'regal' figure made a fascinating impression on her. She was happy to dance with him for an evening. The following evening at dusk she witnessed an outrageous scene—from her window she saw this charming man [*LATIN: fuck a woman in the manner of beasts during menstruation*].*

*[*LATIN: At the sight of running blood and of the man's, as it were, bestial lust*], Miss X. felt completely horrified, as if destroyed, had difficulty regaining her mental equilibrium, was sleepless and lost her appetite for a while and from then on saw in the man the epitome of meanness.*

Two years later, a young lady approached her in a public garden, smiled at her and cast a very peculiar glance at her that penetrated deep into her soul.

The following day, X was driven to visit this park again. The lady was already there and seemed to be waiting for her. They greeted each other like old, dear acquaintances, chatted, joked, and rendezvous were kept daily anew, which continued in the young lady's boudoir when the season became unfavourable. Miss X. reports in her Confidences:]

One day, she led me to her divan, and while she sat down, I let myself slide to her feet. She fixed her shy eyes on me, brushed the hair from my forehead and said: 'Oh, if only I could love you so properly for once. May I?' I said yes, and as we sat there, gazing into each other's eyes, we slid over into the current where there is no turning back. It was captivatingly beautiful; if only I could have painted a picture to immortalise these manifestations. For me, all this was new and intoxicating; one gave oneself up, fully and completely, uninhibited in the most ardent intoxication of female sensuality. I do not think that a man ever matches the enchanting intoxication, the delicate and piquant—men are not refined enough, not sensitive enough. Our wild game had lasted until I sank back exhausted, powerless, enervated. I was lying on her bed, asleep from this exhaustion, when suddenly an unspeakable, unprecedented feeling made me suddenly rise up—a shiver ran through my whole body—I saw J. on top of me—[*LATIN: performing cunnilingus*]—it was the highest pleasure for her [*LATIN: just to be permitted to stare at her breasts*]—whereby she went into convulsive spasms every time.

Thus did our untroubled relationship last for a year, until the transfer of my beloved's father to another town took place.

[KRAFFT-EBING: Miss X. also confessed that during this homosexual intercourse she always felt like a man in relation to the woman and that, [FRENCH: for lack of something better*], she once allowed one of her worshippers to engage in cunnilingus.]*

Notes

1. This term relates to Messalina, who was the third wife of the emperor Claudius and known as a strong and highly promiscuous woman.
2. Hysteropathy is a general term for any of a number of uterine diseases.
3. Aspasia was the consort of the Athenian statesman and general Pericles, renowned as a sexually free courtesan.

CHAPTER 7

Gender Nonconformity

7.1 PS5 (1890) Bb 101, 213–20

R: *PS6 (1891) Bb 106, PS7 (1892) Bb 131, PS8 (1893) Bb 131, PS9 (1894) Bb 127, PS10 (1898) Bb 138, PS11 (1901) Bb 162*

[KRAFFT-EBING: Gynandria. Medical history. On 4 November 1889, the father-in-law of a Count V. reported that the latter had elicited 800 gilders from him under the pretext of needing a bond as secretary of a joint-stock company. Furthermore, it had turned out that Sandor had forged contracts, had faked the marriage ceremony that had taken place in the spring of 1889 and, above all, that this alleged count was not a man at all, but a woman walking around in men's clothing and was called Countess Sarolta (Charlotte) V.

S. was arrested and brought under preliminary investigation for the crime of fraud and forgery of public documents. In the first interrogation, S., born on 6 December 1866, confessed that she was of the female gender, Catholic, unmarried and employed as a writer under the name Count V.

The following remarkable facts, confirmed by other sources, emerge from the autobiography of this female.

S. comes from an old noble, highly respected family in which eccentricity was a family trait. One of her maternal grandmother's sisters was hysterical, a somnambulist who lay in bed for 17 years because of imaginary paralysis. A

D. Pretsell, *Queer Voices in the Works of Richard von Krafft-Ebing, 1883–1901*, Genders and Sexualities in History,
https://doi.org/10.1007/978-3-031-17331-8_7

second great-aunt spent seven years in bed because of an imaginary deathly illness, but still held dances. A third had the quirk that a console in her drawing room was cursed. If someone put something on this console, she became extremely agitated, screamed 'cursed, cursed' and hurried with the object into a room which she called the 'black chamber' and whose key she never let out of her hands. After the death of this lady, a number of shawls, jewellery, banknotes, etc. *were found in the black chamber. A fourth great-aunt did not sweep her room or wash or comb her hair for two years. Only after two years did she reappear. All these women were also witty, educated and kind.*

S.'s mother was nervous and could not stand the moonlight. The paternal family is said to have one spur too many. One line of the family deals almost exclusively with spiritualism. Two blood relatives on the father's side have shot themselves. The majority of the male members are exceptionally talented. The females are all limited, home-baked personalities. S.'s father had a high position, from which he had to resign because of his eccentricity and wastefulness (he squandered over a million and a half).

One of his father's whims was that he raised S. as a boy, made her ride, drive and hunt, admired her energy as a man and called her Sandor. On the other hand, this foolish father had his second son dressed as a woman and brought up as a girl. The farce ended at the age of 15, when this son entered a higher educational institution.

Sarolta-Sandor remained under her father's influence until the age of 12, when she went to Dresden to live with her eccentric maternal grandmother, who, when male sport became too prevalent, took her to an institute and put her into women's clothing. At the age of 13, she entered into a love affair with an Englishwoman, to whom she declared herself to be a boy, and abducted her.

*Sarolta was returned to her mother, who did nothing about it and had to allow her daughter to become Sandor again, to wear boys' clothing and to have at least one love affair with persons of her own sex every year. In addition, S. received a careful education, went on long journeys with her father, naturally always as a young gentleman, emancipated herself early, visited cafés, even ambiguous bars, and even boasted one day at the brothel [*LATIN: girls perched on both knees*]. S. was often intoxicated, passionate about male sports, a very skilled fencer. S. was very attracted to actresses or other single, possibly not quite young ladies. She asserts that she never felt any inclination towards a young man and felt an increasing aversion to men from year to year.]*

I preferred to go with unattractive, inconspicuous men in ladies' company, so that no one would outshine me. If I noticed that one of them aroused sympathy in the ladies, I became jealous. When it came to ladies, I preferred the witty to the physically beautiful. I couldn't stand fat ones or even those who were addicted to men. I loved it when a woman's passion revealed itself under a poetic veil. Everything shameless about a woman was disgusting to me. I had an unspeakable idiosyncrasy against female dresses, against everything feminine in general, but only about and on myself, because on the contrary, I was a fan of the fair sex.

[KRAFFT-EBING: For about 10 years, S. lived almost constantly away from her relatives and as a man. She had a lot of liaisons with ladies, travelled with them, wasted a lot of money and ran up debts. In addition, she devoted herself to literary activities and was a valued contributor to two respected magazines in the capital.

Her passion for ladies was very changeable; there was no constancy in love. Only once did such a liaison last three years. It was years ago that S. made the acquaintance of Emma E., who was 10 years older, at G. Castle. She fell in love with this lady, made a marriage contract with her and lived with her for three years as husband and wife in the capital.

A new love, which was to be fatal for S., caused her to break the 'marriage bond' with E. She did not want to leave her. The latter did not want to let go of her. Only with heavy sacrifices did S. buy her freedom from E., who allegedly still considers herself a divorced woman and Countess V.! That S. was also able to arouse passion in other ladies is evident from the fact that when she had grown tired of a Miss D. (before her 'marriage' to E.), after she had spent several thousand guilders with her, D. threatened to shoot her if she did not remain faithful to her.

It was in the summer of 1887, during a stay in a seaside resort, that S. made the acquaintance of a respected civil servant family E. Immediately, S. fell in love with the daughter Marie and found reciprocal love. Her mother and cousin tried to prevent this love affair, but in vain. Throughout the winter, the two lovers corresponded eagerly with each other. In April 1888, 'Count S.' came to visit and in May 1889 he achieved the goal of his wishes when Marie, who in the meantime had given up a job as a teacher, was married in the presence of a friend of her beloved S. in a garden house by a pseudo-priest in Hungary. The marriage certificate was made by S. and her friend. The couple lived happily and joyously and if not for the complaint of the unpleasant father-in-law, this marriage of convenience would probably have lasted for a long time. It is remarkable that S. knew how to completely deceive the bride's family about her true sex during the rather long bridal state.

S. was a passionate smoker and had masculine airs and passions. Her letters and even court notifications reached her under the address 'Count S.', and she also often spoke of having to enlist for military training. The 'father-in-law' hinted that S. knew how to mark her scrotum by stuffing a sackcloth or glove into her trouser pocket (which she later admitted). The father-in-law also once noticed something like an erect member on the future son-in-law (probably a dildo), who also occasionally let slip the remark that she had to wear a jockstrap when riding. In fact, S. wore a bandage around her body, possibly to fasten a dildo. Although S. often had herself shaved as a matter of form, they were nevertheless convinced in the hotel that she was a woman, because the maid found traces of menstrual blood in the laundry (which S. explained as haemorrhoidal) and on the occasion when S. took a bath were convinced of her female sex through the keyhole.

Marie's family makes it believable that she was long deceived about the true sex of her pseudo-husband. The following passage in a letter from Marie to S. dated 26 August 1889 speaks for the incredible naivety and innocence of this unfortunate girl: 'I don't like other people's children, but I would gladly have such a little one with my Sandi—oh, what happiness, my Sandi!' With regard to S.'s spiritual individuality, a large number of existing manuscripts provide desirable information. The writing has the character of firmness and certainty. They are genuinely masculine features. The content is repeated everywhere in the same characteristics: wild unbridled passion, hatred and resistance against everything that confronts the heart thirsting for love and love in return, love with a poetic touch, in which nothing ignoble is touched, enthusiasm for everything beautiful and noble, a sense for science and the fine arts.

Her writings reveal a colossal knowledge of classics in all languages, quotations from poets and prose writers of all countries. It has also been affirmed by experts that S.'s poetic and literary products are not insignificant.

Psychologically remarkable are the letters and writings touching on her relationship with Marie. S., which speak of the bliss that blossomed at M.'s side and express an immense longing to see her adored wife, even if only for a moment. After such humiliation, she only wishes to exchange the cell for the grave. The bitterest pain is the awareness that Marie now also hates her. Hot tears, so many that she could drown herself in them, she cried for her lost happiness. Entire sheets deal with the apotheosis of this love, reminiscences from the time of their first love and acquaintance.

S. complains about her heart, which would not let itself be dominated by any intellect; she expresses outbursts of emotion that one can only feel, but not simulate. Then again outbursts of the wildest passion with the declaration that she cannot live without Marie.]

Your dear, dear voice, this voice at whose sound I will perhaps rise from the grave, whose sound has always been the promise of paradise to me. Your mere presence was enough to relieve my physical and moral suffering. It was a magnetic current, a peculiar power which your being exerted on mine and which I can never fully define. So I stuck to the eternally true definition: I love her because I love her. In the desolate night I had only one star, the star of Marie's love. The star is now extinguished, only the reflection of it is left, the sweet, wistful memory that illuminates even the truly gruesome night of dying with a soft glow, a glimmer of hope. This writing ends with the apostrophe: gentlemen, wise jurists, psychologists and pathologists, judge me! Every step I took was guided by love, every one of my deeds was conditioned by it—God put it in my heart. If He created me this way and no other, is it my fault or is it the eternally unfathomable ways of fate? I trusted in God that one day salvation would come, for my fault was only love itself, which is the foundation, the principle of His teachings, of His kingdom itself.

My God, you merciful, almighty one, you see my anguish, you know how I suffer. Incline yourself to me and stretch out your helping hand to me, where the whole world has already abandoned me. Only God is just. How beautifully this is described by V. Hugo in his *Légendes du siècle* (The Legend of the ages). How sadly picturesque sounds to me Mendelssohn's melody: every night in my dreams I see you.

[KRAFFT-EBING: Although S. knows that none of her writings reach her 'adored pet', she does not tire of writing outbursts of love-pain and love-joy in page-long deifications of Marie's person,]

only to ask for one more bright shining tear, cried on a still bright summer evening, when the lake glows in the evening light like molten gold and the bells of St Anna and Maria-Wörth, merging in harmonious melancholy, proclaim peace and tranquillity—for that poor soul, for that poor heart, which beat for you to the last breath.

[KRAFFT-EBING: Personal Exploration. The first encounter the court doctors had with S. was somewhat of an embarrassment for both parties, for the former because S.'s perhaps somewhat more garishly forced masculine clothing impacted them, for her because she felt she was being marked with the stigma of moral insanity. A not unattractive, intelligent face which, despite a certain delicacy of features and smallness of all parts, had a decidedly masculine air, were it not for the absence of the sorely missed moustache! Even the

court doctors found it difficult to keep in mind that she was a lady, even though she was dressed as a lady, whereas the intercourse with the man Sandor was much more informal, natural and seemingly more correct. The accused also feels this. She immediately becomes more open, more communicative, freer as soon as she is treated like a man.

Despite her affection for the female sex from her earliest years, it was not until her thirteenth year, when the red-haired Englishwoman was abducted from the Dresden Institute, that she claims to have felt the first traces of sexual impulse, which at that time already manifested itself in kisses, primal embraces and touches with voluptuous sensations. Even then, in her dream images, exclusively female figures appeared to her and she had felt, as she has always felt since then, in the situation of a man in voluptuous dreams and occasionally also felt ejaculation.

*She never engaged in solitary or mutual masturbation. She found such things disgusting and not in keeping with the 'dignity of men' (!). She also never let others touch her [*LATIN: on the genitals*], if only because she was concerned about protecting her great secret. Her periods only started at the age of 17 and were always weak and without discomfort. S. visibly recoils at the discussion of menstrual processes, which is something very repugnant to her masculine consciousness and feelings. She acknowledges the pathological nature of her sexual inclinations, but does not wish for anything else, as she feels completely comfortable and happy in this perverse sensation. The idea of sexual intercourse with men disgusts her and she finds it impossible to carry it out.*

Her shamefulness extended to such an extent that she could rather sleep among men than among women. Thus, when she wanted to satisfy a need or change the laundry, she had to ask her cell mate to turn away from the window so that she could not watch her.

When S. occasionally came into contact with this cell mate, a person from the yeast of the people, she felt lustful excitement and had to blush about it. S. even told us, without being asked, that she was overcome by violent fear when she had to be forced back into the unfamiliar women's clothing in the prison cell. Her only consolation was that she was at least given her men's shirt. Remarkable, and indicative of the importance of olfactory sensations in her sex life, is also her report that she occasionally visited and smelled those parts of the sofa where Mary's head used to lie, in order to inhale the smell of her hair from these places with delight. S. is not particularly interested in beautiful or voluptuous women, not even very young ones. She generally places the physical charms of women in second place. She is attracted to those between *the ages of 24 and 30, as if with a 'magnetic' pull. She found her sexual satisfaction exclusively in [*LATIN: the female body*] (never on her own body) in the form of masturbation of the beloved woman or cunnilingus. Occasionally she also used a stocking stuffed with tallow as a dildo. S. makes these declarations only reluctantly, with obvious shame; just as there is never any shamelessness or cynicism in her writings.*

She is religious, has a lively interest in all that is noble and beautiful, except for men, and is very receptive to moral appreciation on the part of others. She deeply regrets that she made Marie unhappy in her passion, finds her sexual feelings perverse and such love of one woman for another morally reprehensible in healthy people. She is highly talented for literary achievements, possesses a rare memory. Her only weakness is her colossal carelessness and the impossibility of dealing sensibly with money and money's worth. However, she is aware of this weakness and asks not to talk about it any further.

S. is 153 cm tall, of delicate bone structure, lean, but strikingly muscular in the chest and thighs. The gait is awkward in women's clothing. Her movements are strong, not unattractive, though more masculine—stiff, ungraceful. She greets you with a strong handshake. The whole appearance is determined, taut, somewhat self-confident. Her gaze is intelligent, her expression somewhat sombre. Feet and hands conspicuously small, stopped at infantile level. Surfaces of the extremities conspicuously hairy, while there is not even a trace of beard hair, despite all shaving experiments. The torso is not at all of female build. The waist is missing. The pelvis is so slender and so little prominent that a line drawn from the armpit to the corresponding knee corresponds to the direction of the straight line and is not pushed inwards by a waist, nor outwards by the pelvis. The skull is slightly oxycephalic and falls short of the average female in all masses by at least 1 cm.

The cranial circumference is 52, the occipital line 24, the parietal line 23, the frontal line 28.5, the longitudinal circumference 30, the medial line 26.5, the longitudinal diameter 17, the maximum width 13, the distance between the auditory canals 12, and the zygomatic processes 11.2 cm. The upper jaw protrudes strongly, its alveolar process overhangs the lower jaw by 0.5 cm. Tooth position not quite normal. The right upper eye tooth has never developed. Mouth conspicuously small. Ears protruding, lobes undifferentiated, disappearing into the skin of the cheeks. Hard palate, narrow, steep. Voice harsh, deep. Mammary glands sufficiently developed, soft, without secretion. Mons veneris covered with dense dark hairs. Genitalia completely female, without trace of hermaphroditic appearance, but at the infantile stage of a 10-year-old girl. The labia majora touch almost completely, the minora have a cockscomb-like shape and prominence over the major ones. The clitoris is small and highly sensitive. Frenulum tender, perineum very narrow, introitus vaginae narrow, mucous membrane normal. Hymen absent (probably congenital), also the carunculae myrtiformes. Vagina so narrow that insertion of a penis would be impossible, moreover highly sensitive. In any case, coitus has not yet taken place. The Uterus can be felt through the rectum about the size of a walnut, it is immobile and retroflective.

The pelvis appears to be narrowed on all sides (dwarf pelvis) with a decidedly male type. The distance of the anterior iliac spines is 22.5 (instead of 26.3), that of the iliac crests 26.5 (instead of 29.3), that of the trochanter 27.7 (31), the external conjugate 17.2 (19–20), therefore presumably the internal 7.7 (10.8). Because of the insufficient width of the pelvis, the position of the thighs is not convergent as in the female, but straight.

The expert opinion proved that S. has a congenital pathological reversal of sexual feeling, which even anthropologically expresses itself in anomalies of body development, due to severe hereditary strain, and that S.'s incriminating actions are due to her pathological and irresistible sexuality.

In this respect, S.'s significant statement:] 'God has given me love in my heart. If he created me like this and not otherwise, am I to blame, or is it the eternally unfathomable ways of fate?' *[KRAFFT-EBING: had every justification.*

The court delivered an acquittal. The 'countess in men's clothing', as the newspapers called her, returned to her native capital and again got herself known as Count Sandor. Her only sorrow is her ruined love affair with her beloved Marie.]

7.2 NF (1890) Bb 11, 63–6

R: NF (1891) Bb 9, PS7 (1892) Bb 119, PS8 (1893) Bb 119

I. Ancestry: I am now in my twenty-second year; I have chosen the study of medicine as my profession, in which I find complete satisfaction. I have only suffered from mild childhood illnesses, while my siblings, who are all still alive and completely healthy, have had to overcome more serious ones. Both my parents are alive, and my father belongs to the learned class. He, like my mother, is, as they say, very nervously overwrought. My father had a lot of brothers and sisters, but all of them, or at least most of them, died very young. My grandparents are no longer alive, and my grandfathers both died very young.

II. My Person: As far as my physical characteristics are concerned, I am of slender build without being particularly handsome; eyes blue, hair brown. Hair and beard according to sex and age. Mammary glands and genitalia are normally developed. My gait is firm, almost ponderous, my posture sloppy. It is noticeable that the width of my pelvis is completely equal to that of the shoulders.

By nature, I am mentally well endowed. My disposition is even called 'happy' on one of my certificates. I passed my examinations with distinction, without wishing to boast of it, and I have an interest in everything that concerns the welfare of mankind, in science, art and industry. It comes with comparative ease for me to postpone the satisfaction of my needs, to be described below, to a convenient time. I deliberately and consciously condemn today's morality, one which compels sexually abnormal persons to commit offences against arbitrary laws, and consider sexual intercourse between two persons of the same sex to be left to the discretion of the individual, without lawmakers having any right to object. From my studies, I have received the most serious suggestions to build up a morality on the basis of Darwinian views according to Carneri's process,[1] which, although it does not correspond to the present one, would be able to elevate man and ennoble him in the sense of the laws of nature.

One would not find many signs of strain in my case. A certain overexcitement is present. What would perhaps be important is an extremely intense dream life, which is generally occupied with indifferent things, never has so-called voluptuous images as its subject, and at the most is occupied with female clothing and the dressing of the same—which for me, however, is a thought of lust. Sometimes, especially up to the age of 16, it often increased to somnambulism, or very often, as it still does now, to talking aloud in my sleep.

My tendencies: The abnormal tendency just mentioned is the basic principle in my sexual feelings. When I dress in female clothing, I feel complete satisfaction. I am overcome by a peculiar sense of calm and well-being that allows me to engage in lighter mental activity. My libido for sexual intercourse is extremely low. I also have a great sense and taste for female handicrafts and have been able to acquire crochet and embroidery without any instruction, and I enjoy practising these skills in secret. I also enjoy other female tasks, such as sewing and so on, so much that even at home, where I keep my inclination completely hidden and guard against practising it, I have often earned the praise of being a good parlour maid through spontaneous activities, a praise of which I am not at all ashamed, but which, on the contrary, fills me with secret pride. I had no desire at all to dance with women; I only liked to dance with my schoolmates, for which our dance lessons gave me the opportunity; but it was only a pleasure when I was allowed to dance as a lady. I will pass over a number of other desires and reveries that seem to have something typical about them, since they look deceptively similar to those communicated in *Psychopathia Sexualis*, for example, the catafalque fantasies of that young officer, ballet costumes and so on. For the rest, my inclinations are not very different from those of my sex. I smoke and drink moderately, love sweets very much and don't care for physical exercise.

III. History of development: After this brief description of my personality, I can proceed to give a developmental analysis of my abnormal nature. As soon as I was able to think for myself to some extent and I was concerned with the difference between the sexes, it was my secret and firm wish to be a girl. I even believed I was one. But when I occasionally saw the same sexual parts in other boys while bathing, the impossibility of my thought came to me. I reduced my wishes and hoped at least to be a hermaphrodite. And since I had a certain shyness about looking more closely at illustrations or descriptions of sexual parts, this hope persisted, although I had plenty of opportunity to pick up such writings, until my studies forced me to look into this matter more closely. During this time, I read all I could learn about hermaphrodites, and when, as newspapers sometimes reported, a person of the female sex had hitherto been brought up male, and by some accident came to be restored to her sex, I longed to take her place. My recognised masculinity put an end to these dreams and filled me with no particular joy at all. I tried to destroy my sex glands by gradual pressure, but the pain soon made me desist. I still yearn for the outward signs of the female sex: a pretty plait, a round breast, a slender waist.

At the age of 12, I had my first opportunity to put on female clothing, and soon in the evenings I began to drape the bedclothes, sheets and so on in the style of female skirts. Later, when I came of age, it was my greatest delight to secretly put on my sisters' clothes, even if for a few minutes, under the constant danger of discovery. To my delight, I was later allowed to take on a female role in a lovers' play, and I am said to have performed my part quite well. Since I have been leading an independent life as a student, I have immediately procured female clothing and underwear, which I keep organised. In the evening, when I can put on one piece after the other, from the corset to the apron and bracelet—safe from discovery—I am completely satisfied and give myself over to a quiet activity, inwardly happy and eager to create. When I get dressed, I tend to have an erection at first, but this never results in ejaculation and soon disappears. Outwardly, too, I try to get even closer to the female sex by styling my hair appropriately and removing my beard, which I would have liked to pull out.

IV. Sexual inclinations: If I am now to proceed to describe my own sexual inclinations, I would first like to point out in general that my sexual maturity occurred normally, which I infer from the pollutions, voice changes and so on. The pollutions still take place regularly, every three weeks, rarely more often. I never feel any sensation of lust during them. I have never practised masturbation; until recently I only knew the name of the thing and had to find out about it by direct enquiry before I could come to my own conclusion. In general, every touch of the erect member is embarrassing and painful to me, without any feeling of desire.

I used to behave very shyly towards women, now calmly, like equals with equals. I was seldom directly excited by a woman in a sexual sense, but when I try to analyse more closely, it seems to me that it was never her person but only her clothes. I fell in love with her clothes, and the thought of wearing them myself was heavenly. So sexual excitement never took place, not even in brothels, where I was dragged along by friends, despite the display of the most lavishness imaginable, including beauty. But friendly feelings filled my heart for the female sex. I imagined that I could stay with them unrecognised, disguised as a woman, and that I could socialise with them and enjoy myself with them. I am most likely to be impressed by girls whose breasts are not yet overdeveloped, especially those with short hair, because they are closest to me and my way of thinking. Once I was lucky enough to find a girl who felt unhappy in her sex. We formed a firm friendship bond with each other and often enjoyed the idea of both of us exchanging our positions for each other. Perhaps it is not inappropriate and unimportant for the characterisation if I share the following: when, a few months ago, the story of a Hungarian countess went through the newspapers,[2] one who had married disguised as a man and felt herself to be a man, I seriously thought of offering myself to her in order to conclude an inverse marriage—I as a woman, she as a man. I have never tried coitus, nor have I ever felt any desire for it. However, since I foresaw that I would lack the necessary erection with a woman, I decided to put on some of her clothes and thought that the expected success would surely come to pass.

As far as my behaviour towards male persons is concerned, it should be emphasised that I cultivated the most intimate friendships during my school years. My heart was happy if it could do a small service to the one I loved. I really adored him with fervour. But on the other hand, in his case I had terrible fits of jealousy and made such a scene at the slightest occasion. For the duration of the enmity, I felt as if I could not live and could not die. When reconciliation took place, I was again the happiest person for a short time. I also tried to make friends with boys, whom I cuddled, gave all kinds of sweets to and would have liked to kiss. Although my love always remained platonic, it was still abnormal. A remark I made unconsciously at the time about an older friend I adored proves this: I loved him so much, I said, that I would like to marry him. Even now, when I have little intercourse, I am easily infatuated with a handsome male figure, with a fine beard and intelligent features. But I have never found an equally minded soul with whom I could completely discover myself in order to be with him as a girlfriend. I never tried to act on my inclinations directly or to commit any imprudence in this respect. In the end, I refrained from visiting museums where naked male bodies were displayed, as my erections, which would then certainly set in, bothered me to the highest degree. I had sometimes silently longed to sleep with a man, and I found the opportunity. I was invited to do so by an older man whom I disliked quite a bit. We slept together; he touched my sexual organs and despite the fact that I disliked his person, I was filled with a supreme feeling of delight. I felt completely given over to him: in a word, I felt like a woman.

If I may add a final remark to what I have said, I would like to state explicitly that although I am aware of my abnormal inclinations, I do not wish to change them. I only long for a time when I can pursue them more comfortably and with less danger of discovery, in order to give myself a pleasure that harms no one.

7.3 NF (1890) Bb 12, 66–79

R: ***PS7 (1892) Bb 99, PS8 (1893) Bb 99, PS9 (1894) Bb 98, PS10 (1898) Bb 108***

Born in 1842, I was for many years the only child of my parents, as most of the other siblings died of infirmity; only in the 1850s did a brother come along who survived; of him later. First to the antecedents.

My paternal grandfather was forced by external circumstances to marry before his twentieth year, was a craftsman, fathered many children, was immensely industrious and lawful, and possessed a contented nature, though through Bible reading he temporarily got into a one-sided spiritual direction, from which my father tore him out by coaxing him; he lived to be about 90 years of age.

His wife, a little older, also lived to be 90, was healthy and spry, but finally fell into old-age dementia. One of her father's brothers worked himself to death; he had a great sexual need, had three wives and three children by all of them; her sisters were all healthy; they are still alive, very old and physically and mentally normal.

My maternal grandfather also lived to be about 90 years of age, was a sculptor and a factory owner, and fell into old-age dementia. His wife, formerly healthy and full of energy, became melancholic in her last pregnancy and remained so until she died of a stomach ailment at the age of about 65. This marriage produced five sons; the eldest, a renowned doctor, died of apoplexy at the age of about 50, the other of typhoid fever, a third fell at the hands of a murderer, a fourth, a popular physician, died of tuberculosis at the age of about 42; the latter was in every respect more than half a woman, painted well, loved fishing, was impotent, but very popular and skilful, not a surgeon, but a good obstetrician; the last, a high official and a man of deep disposition, died of stomach cancer at over 60 years of age; he was honesty and devotion to duty personified.

Of the daughters, the eldest was scrofular, died of dropsy; the second, my mother, also died of dropsy; the third died of typhoid; the fourth is alive, is hysterical; the fifth is about 50 years of age, hysterical and melancholic to the point of mental disorder; the youngest (fifth) had more the character of a boy in her youth and was just as cheerful as she is melancholic now. My mother was anaemic but was especially endowed with great energy and diligence. She gave birth to several children and submitted to my somewhat harsh father with the greatest patience. At the same time, however, she displayed great courage on many occasions and was most willing to make sacrifices for the whole family and, after an earlier period of sentimentality, truly pious to the day she died, a noble and patient person; I only knew her as a moody person during her last pregnancy, when I no longer really knew or understood her.

Now to my brother, he died at the age of 30 after a misspent life. He was graceful, had a sparse beard, quite the figure of a beautiful girl, by which he also had the capriciousness and a certain volatility, but also the goodness and kindness; if he was dressed as a lady, no one recognised him; his whole bearing, manner, everything was genuine; he was then the image of his mother; first educated in a school run by women, he was the rascal of the first kind, and no prank was omitted, yet he was good-natured. As a grammar school pupil, he was a model pupil in terms of knowledge, and as a conscript he was a good soldier who was respected for all his daring pranks. As a student, he unfortunately changed his studies course and occupied himself with social policy; he devoted himself passionately to medicine; here he benefited from his rare skill in drawing and painting; he had a picture of everything in his head and it was always at his disposal within a few moments; he was popular with the sick; his gaze was sure, his scalpel likewise. As a reserve officer he was dashing and popular, but in the service he contracted pleurisy, which was the beginning of his tuberculosis. He thought very highly of his appearance; although not foppish, he possessed a feminine vanity and unfortunately also a feminine fickleness.

Now to my father: In the last years of his life, he suffered from a decreasing ability to express himself, probably as a result of several strokes and constant overwork; for three years, from about the age of 76, he alternated between apathy and agitation. Brought up in poor circumstances, gifted with talents as great as his firmness of will, he studied with distinction first theology, then philosophy and so on and devoted himself with happiness to teaching abroad. In his old age he became mentally disturbed, and in his last years he unfortunately showed unambiguous signs of the highest degree of libido.

Now, unfortunately, I come to myself, and despite the high degree of disgust, I want and must describe myself to you in full.

As a small child, I was said to be very pretty, with blond curls and transparent skin; very obedient, quiet, modest, so that I was taken to every ladies' party without being teased. Judging by my crooked legs, I was not entirely free of rickets. With a very active imagination, my enemy all my life, my talents developed quickly. At the age of four I could read and write—my memory goes back to the third year. I played with everything I could lay my hands on, with lead soldiers or stones or ribbons from a children's shop; only an apparatus for making wood, which was given to me, I did not like. I preferred to be at home with my mother, who was my everything. I had two or three friends, with whom I socialised good-naturedly, but I liked their sisters just as much, who always treated me like a girl, which did not please me at first.

I must have been on the way to becoming like a girl—at least, I remember well how it was always said: 'that is not suitable for a boy'. Then I tried to play the boy, imitated everything my friends did and tried to surpass them in wildness, which I succeeded in doing; no tree or building was too high for me not to climb. I took great pleasure in playing soldiers, but avoided the girls more, as I was not supposed to play with their things, and it always pained me that they treated me so completely as their own.

In the company of adults, however, I was always equally modest and equally welcome. I was often tormented by fantastic dreams of strange animals that once drove me out of bed without me waking up. I was always dressed simply, but in a very dainty way, and this gave me an inclination for beautiful clothing; it seems to me that I have had an inclination for women's gloves since my school days, which I secretly put on as often as I could; so when my mother once gave away a pair of them, I was quite energetically against it and told my mother on questioning that I would have preferred to have them myself. I was laughed at, and from then on I was very careful not to show my preference for female things. And yet my pleasure was so great. I especially enjoyed masquerade dresses, that is, only female ones; when I saw them, I envied the owner. My favourite thing was to see two young gentlemen cross-dressed as powdered ladies, albeit beautifully, with very pretty girls' noses on their faces, and yet I would not have shown myself as a girl in front of others at any price; I was so afraid of being ridiculed. At school I showed the greatest diligence and was always top in the class; my parents taught me from childhood that duty comes first and always gave me an example of this; attending school was also a pleasure for me because the teachers were gentle and the older pupils did not torment the younger ones. Now we left my first home, as my father was forced to separate from the family for a year for the sake of journalism; we moved to Germany. Here, a strict to rough tone prevailed, partly among the teachers, partly among the pupils, and I was ridiculed again because of my girlishness.

My fellow pupils went so far as to give my name to a girl who had exactly my features and hers to me, so that I hated the girl with whom I later became friends when she was married. My mother continued to dress me daintily, and this was repugnant to me, as it always earned me ridicule, so that I was glad when I finally got quite proper trousers and quite proper men's coats. But with these came a new nuisance; they irritated my genitals, especially when the cloth was a little rough, and the touch of the tailor when fitting me was quite unbearable to me because of its tickling sensation, which made me shudder, especially on my genitals. Now I was supposed to do gymnastics and I simply could not do everything or had difficulties around the exercises that girls cannot do easily; when bathing I was plagued by the shame of exposing myself, but I did it very gladly; until the age of 12 I had a great weakness in my lower back. I learned to swim late but was good at it and could swim great distances. At the age of 13 I had pubes, was about 6 feet tall, but in the face, I was a woman until the age of 18, when my beard came in strongly and I was afraid of looking like a woman.

An inguinal hernia, acquired at the age of 12 and not cured until the age of 20, was a great nuisance to me, especially during gymnastics; from the age of 12 onwards, when sitting for long periods of time and especially during night work, which was often long, there was an itching, burning and trembling from my penis to beyond the small of my back, which made sitting and standing difficult and was aggravated when it was cold; however, I had no idea that this could have anything to do with the genitals. Since none of my friends suffered from it, it seemed quite strange to me, and I needed the utmost patience to endure it, all the more so because my abdomen often annoyed me.

I was still completely ignorant about sexual matters, but now, at the age of 12 or 13, I had the certain feeling that I would rather be a woman. I liked her figure better, her calm demeanour, her decency, but especially her clothing was very appealing to me. I was careful not to let it be noticed, but I know for certain that I would not have shied away from the castration knife in order to achieve my goal. If I had had to say why I preferred to dress in women's clothing, I could only have said that I was drawn to them by force; perhaps I also felt more like a girl because of my unusually soft skin, which was very sensitive, especially on my face and hands. I liked to be seen with girls; although I would have preferred to be among them all the time, I mocked them wherever I could, for I had to exaggerate in order not to appear effeminate myself, and yet I always envied them in my heart; my envy was especially great when a friend got long dresses and walked in gloves and veils. When I was 15 and on a journey, a young lady with whom I was staying suggested that I masquerade as a lady and go out with her; but, as she was not alone, I did not accept, much as I would have liked to. That was how little trouble I was put to; I was pleased to see on that journey that the boys in a town wore blouses with short sleeves and bare arms. A very clean lady seemed like a goddess to me; if I touched her ice-cold hand, I was happy and envious, and would have loved to be in her place in her beautiful clothes and delicate figure. Nevertheless, I studied very diligently, completed secondary school and grammar school in nine years, and passed a good school-leaving examination. I remember expressing the 'wish to be a girl' to a friend for the first time at the age of 15; I could not answer his question as to why.

By the age of 17, I was in easy company, I drank a lot of beer, smoked and tried to joke with waitresses; they liked to socialise with me, but they always treated me as if I wore skirts. I couldn't go to dance class; they drove me out; if I could have gone in disguise, it would have been different. I loved my friends tenderly, only one I hated, who had tempted me into onanism. Fie on that day, which damaged me for life. I pursued it quite often but felt like a double man in the process. I can't describe the feeling; I think it was masculine but mixed with feminine. I couldn't get close to a girl. I feared them and yet they were not alien to me; but they impressed me more than someone like me would. I envied them; I would have renounced all pleasures if I had been allowed to be a girl at home after class and if I had been allowed to go out like that; a crinoline, a skimpy glove was just my ideal. Every time I saw a lady's suit, I felt how it would make me feel, namely, as a lady; I had no longing to be a man.

I do remember being quite fond of a beautiful male friend who had a girl's face and dark curls, but I think I only had the wish that we could both become girls.

At college, I finally got to coitus once, but didn't have a much different feeling than that I would have preferred to be on the bottom and would have gladly swapped my penis with her vagina. The girl also, to her surprise, had to treat me like a girl, which she gladly agreed to, but also treated me as if I were now she (she was still pretty stupid and didn't mock me for it).

As a student, I was wild at the time, but always felt that I was only putting on this wildness as a mask; I drank, picked fights, but could not take dance lessons again because I was afraid of betraying myself. My friendships were intimate, but without ulterior motives; I was most pleased when a friend masqueraded as a lady or when I could examine the ladies' makeup at a ball; I had every understanding for this and gradually began to feel like a woman.

Due to unfortunate circumstances, I made two suicide attempts; once, for no reason, I did not sleep for 14 days, had many hallucinations (sight and hearing at the same time), and communicated with the dead and the living at the same time, which has remained with me to this day.

I also had a girlfriend who knew about my love affair, who put on my gloves, but who also only regarded me as a girl. So I understood women better than any other man, and when they realised that, I behaved like a woman, as though they had a girlfriend. On the whole, I couldn't stand it when I was propositioned, and actually only went along with it for bragging sake when it happened. I soon got over my initial disgust at the odour of blood, but I could never see individual things without disgust. Only one thing was always lacking in me, that I was always uncertain about myself; I knew that I had feminine inclinations, but still believed I was a man, but I doubt whether—apart from coitus attempts which never gave me pleasure (which I attributed to masturbation)—I ever once admired a woman without the desire to be the same, or to ask myself whether I would like to be her or appear in her finery. In midwifery, which I found very difficult to learn (I was embarrassed for the girls lying down and felt sorry for them), I have to this day had to overcome a feeling of horror; indeed, it has happened to me that I felt as if I were feeling the tractions. Having successfully served in several places as a medical assistant, I took part in a campaign as an assistant doctor and staff doctor. Riding, which I was already embarrassed about as a student because my genitals conveyed more feminine feelings, was difficult for me (it would have been easier in a woman's way).

I still believed I was a man with uncertain feelings, and whenever I came into contact with ladies, I was soon treated as a uniformed lady instead (when I wore the uniform for the first time, I would much rather have slipped into a lady's costume with a veil; it was a disturbing feeling for me when people looked at the handsome uniformed man). In private practice, I was lucky in all three main branches. Then I went on another campaign. In this one, my nature came in handy, as I don't think any animal since the first donkey in the world has had to show as much patience as I have. Decorations were not absent, but they left me cold.

So I made my way through life as best I could, never satisfied with myself, full of world-weariness, wavering between sentimentality or wildness, which was mostly affectation.

As a marriage candidate, I was in a very peculiar situation. I would have preferred not to marry at all, but family circumstances and practice forced me to do so. I married an energetic, amiable lady from a family where female domination flourished. I was in love with her, as well as I could be, that is, what one loves, he loves with all his heart and is absorbed in it, even if he does not appear as ardent as a whole and genuine man; he loves his bride with all feminine depth, almost like a bridegroom, only I did not admit this side to myself, because I still believed that I was just a disgruntled man who would probably come to himself and find himself through marriage. But already on the wedding night, I felt that I was only functioning as a woman in male form; I would rather have had my place on the bottom. On the whole, we lived happily and contentedly, remaining childless for a few years. After a difficult pregnancy, during which I lay dead tired in enemy territory, a difficult birth was followed by the first boy, to whom a melancholy nature still clings today; then a second, who is quite calm; a third full of pranks; a fourth; a fifth; all of them already have a predisposition to neurasthenia. As I never felt at home, I went out a lot in cheerful company, but always worked as hard as a man could, studied, operated, experimented with many medicines and cures, and also always on myself. In marriage, I left the running of the house to my wife, as she is very good at keeping house. I performed my duties as a husband as well as I could, but without satisfaction for me; from the first coitus until today, the male position has been repugnant and too difficult for me. I would much rather have had the other role. When I had to help my wife give birth, it almost broke my heart, because I empathised with her pain. We lived together for a long time until severe gout drove me into various baths and finally made me neurasthenic. At the same time, I became so anaemic that every few months I had to take iron for a while, otherwise I was chlorotic or hysterical, or both together. Stenocardia often plagued me, then came hemiplegic cramps in the chin, nose, throat, larynx, hemicrania, spasms of the diaphragm and pectoral muscles; for about three years I felt as if my prostate were enlarged, with a feeling of expulsion, as if I were to give birth to something, pains in the hip, perennial backache and so on; but I defended myself with the fury of despair against these complaints that impressed me as feminine or female, until three years ago a very violent attack of arthritis broke me completely. Even before this terrible attack of gout occurred, in desperation to eradicate the gout, I took hot baths, as close to body heat as possible. It happened once that I suddenly felt changed and close to death; I jumped out of the bath with the last of my strength, but had felt completely like a woman with libido. Furthermore, at the time when extract of *Cannabis indica* came into use and was even praised, I took about three to four times the usual dose out of fear of my impending gout attack (and tormented by indifference to life) and underwent a life-and-death hashish intoxication. Laughing spasms, a feeling of unheard-of physical strength and speed, my own feeling in my brain and eyes, billions of sparks from my brain flashing through my skin set in, but I could still force myself to speak; all at once I saw myself as a woman from my toes to my chest, felt, as before in the thermal baths, that my genitals were pushed inwards, my pelvis widened, my breasts shot out, and an unspeakable lust took hold of me. Then I closed my eyes, so that at least I didn't see my face change. My doctor looked as if he had a giant potato instead of a head, my wife had a full moon on her torso. And yet, when they both left the room for a short time, I was strong enough to write a short last will in my notebook.

But who can describe my horror when I awoke the next morning, feeling completely transformed into a woman, and felt a vulva and breasts as I walked and stood? When I finally got out of bed, I felt that a whole change had taken place in me. Even during the illness, a visitor said, 'for a man he is so patient' and gave me a flowering vine as a gift, which alienated me but made me happy! From then on, I was patient, no longer wanted to do anything in a storm, but became as tough as a cat, but at the same time mild, conciliatory, no longer retrospective: in short, like a woman in her own image. During the last illness, I had many visual and auditory hallucinations, spoke with the dead and so on, saw and heard familiar spirits and felt like a double person, but I did not yet notice in my sickbed that the man in me had gone out. My change of mood was fortunate, as I was struck by a blow that would have killed me in my former mood, but which I now accepted with surrender, so that I no longer recognised myself. As I often mistook the symptoms of neurasthenia for gout, I continued to take many baths until a skin itch with the sensation of scabies increased instead of diminishing, so that I gave up all external therapy (I came to feel more and more anaemic from the baths) and hardened myself as best I could. But the feminine compulsion remained and became so strong that I only wear the mask of a man, but otherwise feel in every respect to be a perfect woman in all parts and have lost all memory of the old times. What the gout had left was completely ruined by the influenza.

Present Status: I am over 6 feet tall, my hair has thinned out, I have lost my teeth, my beard is turning grey, my posture is beginning to come to a stoop; since the influenza I have lost about a quarter of my raw strength. Face looks somewhat reddened as a result of a valvular defect; full beard; chronic conjunctivitis; more muscular than fat; left foot seems to get varicose veins, falls asleep often, is not yet visibly thickened, but seems to become so.

My mammillary region stands out clearly in spite of smallness. My abdomen has the shape of a woman's belly, feet placed after a woman's manner, calves and so on; with my arms it is just so and with my hands. Can wear women's stockings and gloves 7 ¾ 7 ½; likewise, I wear a corset without complaint. Weight alternates between 168 and 184 pounds.

Urine without protein, without sugar, contains uric acid above the norm; but if it does not contain much uric acid, it is light, almost watery after any excitement of any kind. Stool usually regular, but if it is not, all the female complaints of constipation are present. Sleep poor, often for many weeks only two to three hours. Appetite quite good, but on the whole my stomach cannot bear more than that of a strong woman and reacts immediately to sharp food by skin rash and burning in the urethra. Skin is white, on the whole it feels very smooth; intolerable itching in it for two years, has diminished in the last few weeks, only shows more in the hollow of my knee and on my scrotum.

Tendency to perspiration; sweat, formerly almost non-existent, now undergoes all the ugly nuances of female sweat, especially on the lower body, so that I have to keep myself even cleaner than a woman (perfume the handkerchief, use of perfumed soaps and cologne).

General feeling: I feel like a woman in the shape of a man. Even if I sometimes still feel the shape of a man, the respective member still feels feminine, for example, the penis as clitoris; the urethra as urethra and vaginal orifice, it always feels a little wet, even if it is still so dry; the scrotum as labia majora; in short, I always feel a vulva and only those who feel or have felt like this themselves know what this means. But the whole skin of my whole body feels feminine, takes in all impressions, whether they be those of touch, warmth or hostile ones, as a woman, and I have the sensations of one; I cannot go out with bare hands, for heat and cold both torment me very much; when the time when we gentlemen are allowed to carry the parasol has passed, I have to suffer very great pain in my facial skin until the parasol may come to be used again. When I wake up in the morning, it dawns on me for a few moments, it is as if I am looking for myself, then the compulsive feeling of being a woman awakens; I feel the sensation of the vulva (or that there is one) and greet the day with a silent or loud sigh, for I am already afraid of the dramas to come all day. It is no small thing to feel like a woman and have to act like a man. I had to learn everything anew; the knives, the apparatus, everything has felt completely different since three years ago, and with the changed muscle feeling, I had to learn everything anew. I succeeded—only the guidance of the saw and the bone chisel is still a problem for me; it is almost as if the brute strength was not quite sufficient. On the other hand, I have more feeling when working with the sharp spoon in the soft parts; it is sickening that when examining ladies, I often feel their feelings, which does not alienate them. The most unsavoury thing I feel is a child's movement. For a time, several months,

I was tormented by the reading of thoughts in both sexes, against which I still have to fight; with women I can bear it more easily, with men it is repugnant to me. Three years ago, I did not yet consciously look at the world with female eyes; this change in the response of the optic centre of the brain came almost suddenly with a severe headache. I was with a lady who felt sexually inverted, and suddenly I saw her so changed as I now feel, namely, that she was a man and that I felt myself to be a woman towards her, that I left her with ill-concealed anger; at that time, she had not yet come to realise her condition.

Since then, all my senses make their perception in female form and likewise their response. The cerebral system was almost immediately joined by the vegetative system, so that all complaints manifested themselves in a feminine way: the sensitivity of all nerves, especially of the acusticus, olfactorius or trigeminus, increased to nervousness. If only a window flaps, I collapse, that is, inwardly—what to the man is not allowed; if a dish is not absolutely fresh, I have the smell of cadaver in my nose. I would never have thought the trigeminal system capable of such capricious pain jumping from one branch to the next, from one tooth to the eye.

But since my change, I can bear toothache and migraine more easily, and I also have less anxiety when I have stenocardia. It seems to be a peculiar observation that I feel like a fearful, weaker being, but that I am much more cold-blooded and calmer in the face of imminent danger, and also during very difficult operations. My stomach takes revenge for the slightest mistake (against a woman's diet) in a woman's way, be it through ructus or other complaints, especially alcohol abuse. The hangover of a man who feels like a woman is much more infamous than the most colossal college hangover; it almost seems to me as if, feeling like a woman, one is completely under the control of the vegetative system.

As small as my nipples are, they want space and I feel them as mammaries, just as the nipples were already swollen and painful in puberty; that's why every white shirt, waistcoat and coat irritates me. Of the pelvis I have the feeling as if it were a feminine one, ditto of the anus and nates [buttocks]; disturbing to me in the beginning was the feeling of femininity of the belly, which does not want to fit into any trousers and always produces or possesses the feeling of femininity. I also have the compulsive feeling of a waist. I feel as if, deprived of my own skin, I were put into a woman's skin, which adapts itself exactly to everything, but feels everything as if it surrounded a woman, including the feelings that flow through the whole enclosed man's body and exude the male ones. My testicles, although not atrophic or degenerated, are no longer testicles and often cause me pain with the impression that they belong in the abdomen and should be stuck there; their mobility often torments me.

Every four weeks, at the time of the full moon, I have all the symptoms of a period for five days, like a woman, physically and mentally, except that I do not bleed, while I have a feeling of discharge of fluid, a feeling of swelling of the genitals and the abdomen (inside); a very pleasant time, especially when afterwards and later for a few days in the meantime the physiological feeling of needing to be mated comes with its whole, woman-pervading power; my whole body is then full of this feeling, like a dipped piece of sugar is sucked full of water or as full as a wet sponge. There it is said: first woman in need of love, then man, and indeed the need, as it seems to me, is more a longing for conception than for coitus. The immense natural instinct or female desire, however, makes the sense of shame recede, so that coitus is indirectly desired. I have felt coitus as a man at most three times in my life, if at all, and indifferently in all other cases; in the last three years, however, I have felt it distinctly passively as a woman, even sometimes with a female feeling of ejaculation; I always feel mated and fatigued like a woman, often also uncomfortable, as a man never feels. Sometimes it has caused me such great pleasure that I can compare it with nothing else; it is simply the most blissful, most powerful feeling on earth, for which everything can be sacrificed; at that moment the woman is only vulva, which has devoured the whole person.

I have not lost the feeling of being a woman for a moment in three years; now, through habituation, it is no longer so embarrassing to me, although since then I feel inferior, for to feel womanly without a desire for pleasure is bearable even for a man; but when needs come! Then the pleasure ceases; the burning, the warmth, the turgor feeling of the genitals (when the penis is not erect, the genitals fall out as if from the role). A sensation of desire that occurs during strong urges in the vagina and vulva is downright horrible, a hellish torment of lust, but hardly endurable. If I am then in a position to perform coitus, it is better, but because of the lack of conception it does not bring full and constant satisfaction; the feeling of sterility sets in with all its shameful pressure, along with the feeling of passive mating, the injured sense of shame; one almost feels like a lustful whore. Reason is of no help—the compulsive feeling of femininity dominates and conquers everything. It is easy to imagine how difficult it is to work professionally in such times, but one can force oneself to do so. Admittedly, it is almost impossible to sit, walk, lie down; at least none of these three states can be endured for long, plus the constant touching of the trousers and so on is unbearable.

Marriage then, apart from the moment of coitus, when the man must feel himself mated, still gives the impression of the cohabitation of two women, one of whom regards herself as a husband in the masculine sense. If these periodic molimina[3] are once absent, then come the feelings of gravidity or sexual satiety, which the man does not otherwise know, but which take hold of the whole man just as the feeling of womanhood does, only that these feelings are specifically repulsive, so that one gladly puts up with the regular period again. When erotic dreams or imaginings come, one sees oneself in the form one would have as a woman and sees erect members that present themselves; since the anus also feels feminine, it would not be at all difficult to become the passive sodomite; only the positive religious prohibition prevents it, and all other considerations would become invalid.

Since such conditions will probably come to everyone as repugnant, there is a longing to be sexless or to be allowed to make oneself sexless. If I were single, I would have long since bid farewell to testicles and scrotum along with penis.

What is the use of the highest female feeling of pleasure if one does not conceive? What use are the impulses of female love, if one seeks sexual satisfaction with a woman and that mating makes one feel like a man? How horribly shameful is the female perspiration! How degrading to the man is the feeling of pleasure in dresses and jewellery! Even in the transformed form, even if he can no longer remember the male sexual feeling, he does not want to have to feel like a woman; he still knows quite well that in former times he did not always feel sexual, that he was also a mere human being, uninfluenced by sex! Now, all of a sudden, he is supposed to feel that his previous individuality is only a mask, that he always feels like a woman, that he only has a change when he has his periodic complaints every four weeks and his female, unsatisfiable lust time in between? When will he be allowed to wake up without immediately having to feel like a woman? Finally, he longs for a moment when he could lift his mask, but the moment does not come! He can only find relief from his misery if he can put on a piece of womanhood, jewellery, an undergarment and so on, for he is not allowed to walk as a woman after all; to have to fulfil all his professional duties with the feeling of an actress costumed as a gentleman and to foresee no end to it is no small matter. Religion alone protects against gross lapses but does not prevent the embarrassment when the temptation comes to the female-feeling individual as it does to a real woman and must be felt and gone through in this way! When a respected man, who enjoys rare public confidence and authority, has to struggle with his vulva, even if it is imaginary; when one comes from a hard day's work and is compelled to examine the appearance of the nearest lady, to criticise her with a woman's eyes, to read her thoughts from her face; when a fashion journal (which I already had as a child) inspires the same interest as a scientific work? When you have to hide your condition from your wife, whose thoughts, as soon as you feel like a woman, you have to hide from your face, while it comes to her that you have changed in body and soul. The torment caused by the feminine softness that has to be overcome! It is true that sometimes, when one is alone on holiday, one succeeds in living more like a woman for a while, for example, in wearing female dresses and so on, especially at night. But femininity, once invaded, comes to demand imperiously that it be acknowledged; it is often content with a modest concession, for example, the wearing of a bracelet behind the cuff, but it demands imperiously a concession of some kind. The only happiness is that one can see oneself in female costume without shame. Indeed, if one's face is veiled or masked, one prefers to see oneself that way and to feel natural, then, like any other fashion goose, one has the taste of the current fashion, so much is one transformed! Until one has become accustomed to the idea of feeling independently only as a woman, and of bringing the former way of thinking, as it were, only from memory for comparison, then expressing oneself as a man takes a long time and unspeakable conquest.

Nevertheless, it will still happen that one catches oneself in a feminine expression of feeling, be it in sexuality, that one says: one feels this way and that way, which, however, a non-female cannot know, or that one accidentally reveals that female clothing is commonplace.

In front of women alone this makes no difference, since a woman feels flattered in the first place if one understands something about her things, only it must not happen in front of one's own wife! How shocked I was once when my wife told a friend that I had a very refined taste in women's articles! How surprised a haughty fashionable lady was when I explained to her, who was about to bring up her little daughter all wrong, all female feelings in writing and orally (I lied to her that I had drawn my knowledge from letters); but just as great is her confidence now, and the child, on the way to becoming insane, has remained sensible and is cheerful. For she had confessed all the stirrings of womanhood as sins; now she knows what she must endure as a girl and master by will and religion and feels herself to be a person. The two ladies would laugh heartily if they knew that I have only drawn from my own sad experience. I must add that since then I have a much finer feeling for temperature, and in addition a feeling for the elasticity of the skin, for tension of the intestines and so on in patients, which was unknown to me before, but that during operations and dissections hostile fluids penetrate my (uninjured) skin more easily. Every dissection causes me pain, every examination of a prostitute or a woman with fluorine, or the smell of cancer and so on affects me in a downright hostile way. In general, I am now strongly influenced by antipathy and sympathy, from the sense of colour to the judgement of a whole person. Women usually see each other's present sexual mood, which is why a lady wears a veil, even if she doesn't always wear it, and usually wears perfume, even if it is only a handkerchief or gloves, because her sense of smell towards her sex is enormous; in general, smells have an incredible effect on a female organism; for example, violets and roses calm me, while other smells disgust me—with ylang-ylang I couldn't stand it because of sexual excitement. Touching a woman seems homogeneous to me, coitus with a woman seems possible to me if she is a little more masculine, has a firm skin, and yet it is more like lesbianism.

Moreover, I always feel passive. When I often can't sleep at night because I'm so excited, it finally works if I keep my legs apart like a woman doing a nude, or lie down on one side, but then no arm or part of the bed may touch my breast, otherwise it's over again with sleep; also my stomach doesn't like to be pressed. I sleep best in a woman's shirt and bed jacket, and then with gloves, because my hands freeze easily; I also like to sleep in women's underwear and petticoats, because they don't touch my genitals. I liked women's clothing best at the time of the crinolines. Women's dresses do not irritate the feminine-feeling person, because he feels them, like every woman, as belonging to his person, not as foreign objects.

My favourite social intercourse is with a lady suffering from neurasthenia, who has felt male since the last postpartum bed, but who, since I have explained these feelings to her, has been doing her best to abstain from coitus—which I, as a man, am not allowed to do: she helps me to bear my condition by her example. She remembers women's feelings even more clearly and has already given me some good advice. If she were a man and I a young girl, I would try to acquire her, before her I would put up with a woman's fate. But her present photograph is quite different from the earlier ones; she is a most elegantly costumed gentleman in spite of bosom and so on and hairdo; but she also speaks briefly and succinctly, and no longer takes any pleasure in anything that amuses me; she has a kind of world-weariness, but bears her fate with surrender and dignity, finds her consolation only in religion and the fulfilment of duty, almost goes to pieces at the time of her menses; she no longer loves women's company and women's conversation, nor sweets.

A male friend of my youth has felt since the first time of life only as a girl but has affection for the male sex; his sister had it the other way round, and when the uterus demanded its right and she saw herself as a loving woman, despite her maleness, she cut it short and took her own life by drowning.

The main changes I have observed in myself since complete effemination are:

1. the constant feeling of being a woman from the top of my head to my toes,
2. the constant feeling of possessing female genitalia,
3. the periodicity of the monthly menses,
4. the regular occurrence of female desire, but without lust for a particular man,
5. during coitus, a female passive feeling,
6. afterwards the feeling of the sexually receptive party,
7. at pictures of coitus, the female feeling,
8. at the sight of women's rooms, the feeling of togetherness and the female interest in it,
9. at the sight of gentlemen, the female interest in them,
10. at the sight of children, the same,
11. the change of temper, the much greater patience,
12. the final successful surrender to my fate, which I owe only to positive religion, otherwise I would long since have given up.

For to be a man and to have to feel [*FRENCH: every woman is the fucked or she desires to be*] is hardly bearable.

Notes

1. Bartholomäus von Carneri, Austrian philosopher who wrote on materialist ethics based on Darwinism.
2. This is a reference to Count Sandor, the passing man in the previous case study – 7.1.
3. 'Molimina' is an old medical term for premenstrual sensations.

CHAPTER 8

Pathologisers

8.1 PS3 (1888) Bb 32, 77–80

One day, in the privy of the grammar school, while I was looking unsuspectingly into the eyes of my comrade, he handed me his erect penis with the request '[*LATIN: put my penis in your mouth*]'. I indignantly rejected this request, hated the most beautiful man for a moment because of this mean imposition, but soon the longing for him, for his beautiful whole body, returned and awakened powerful erections in me. One evening, as I pined for him in my thoughts, the most beautiful man approached me, touched my [*LATIN: genitals*] while at the same time masturbating himself. I fled, but on the same day I could no longer restrain myself from the sexual excitement of masturbating [*LATIN: my genitals*]. There, under indescribably sweet feelings, in thoughts of clinging to the mouth of the most beautiful man, close to fainting, I had my first ejaculation. I was 15 years of age at the time. My inclination for that young man, my raging love for him lasted for several years. I never granted his wishes, but in the ecstasy of the thought, lying firmly on him in my imagination, I often satisfied myself by masturbating.

From the age of 17 onwards, I spent a lot of time in the company of ladies and at balls, danced passionately, but never had a feeling of affection in the presence of a lady, even the most beautiful one—on the contrary, when ladies flirted with me, as was the case, for example, at the ladies' ball,

D. Pretsell, *Queer Voices in the Works of Richard von Krafft-Ebing, 1883–1901*, Genders and Sexualities in History,
https://doi.org/10.1007/978-3-031-17331-8_8

I was silently enraged. This kindness disgusted me; it seemed so disgustingly mean to me—and yet I would have liked to dance passionately and in a feminine manner with some of my teachers. I was particularly attracted to one of them by his physique and promising appearance. For a while, I had the most ardent wish to be the lover of this 45-year-old man.

I deliberately arranged it in such a way that I committed minor school misdemeanours and therefore had to come to his apartment. I trembled with delight when I heard his footsteps. I was plagued with such desires and cravings towards other beloved students for years. I fell in love with a medical student, went on long journeys with him at my own expense so that I could have him with me all the time, celebrated him with the most ardent poems and was often almost sensually drunk, loving him in my thoughts. My sense of honour, my moral consciousness prevented me from having anything but the most decent dealings with him. Nevertheless, that time was the most beautiful of my life, even though I almost pined away in longing for love and spent many a sleepless night. At the time, I satisfied myself by thinking of myself at the side of these dear people. In order to get to know me, I suppose, this friend took me to a brothel one evening.

The situation was terrible for me there. I was greatly comforted by the fact that the friend was content to converse there. One day he dropped the word 'urning' and gave me an explanation. I was horrified by this, for I considered love of one's own sex to be immorality, a thing deserving contempt. Violent anguish of soul arose from the consciousness that, in spite of moral education and the best of wills, I could never tread the natural path. I became all the sadder and more unhappy as I approached mature manhood, having the desire to establish a family life at all costs, which was the only ideal life I had in mind from my parents' home. This was the beginning of a difficult time for me. I had never felt the slightest inclination towards a female being!

My hope was to learn to feel differently towards a girl who captivated me with her spiritual advantages. On the other hand, I had more and more the suspicion that my feelings were based on a natural predisposition, especially since the urge to desire a handsome, strong man, which I had fought down with all my energy, was constantly reappearing.

I shuddered at the thought of not being able to achieve my ideal life, the happiness of a family life. I travelled through half of Europe, avoided men in every country, often ideally beautiful ones, who approached me with desire and whom I would have liked to embrace and kiss if my sense of honour had allowed it. When I returned home, I had to take over my family's estate. In the loneliness of country life, the desire for a family life became overpowering. I found a girl who was equally outstanding in spirit and mind, entered into a pure marriage of convenience at the age of 30 and went to the altar with a childlike, joyful spirit, hoping that with this lovely creature my love for men would disappear without a trace and that I would become quite happy. The opposite happened. I was deeply unhappy as often as I thought of a certain duty, and only with the greatest overcoming, out of compassion for my adored and beloved wife, with the help of the imagination, in the thought of a beautiful male figure that I liked, did I manage to achieve erection, to fulfil my duty and to produce two healthy and happy children. I suffered immeasurably physically and morally in conjugal intercourse with my wife, while a pleasant male figure could cause me the most violent erection, the most ardent desire and at times put me in the absolute necessity to masturbate.

For the past year I have been completely impotent towards my beloved wife, while attractive men excite me to the highest degree and make me pine for a pleasure that my sense of honour forbids me to achieve.

Since I know that many men feel the same way I do and allow themselves the satisfaction of their urges, my desire is even stronger than before. I suffer physically and morally in agony, feel that my nerves are coming to pieces and that I will wear myself out. I have done everything possible to protect myself from excitement, for example, exchanged all male domestics whom I liked to ones I didn't like and so on.

[KRAFFT-EBING: The patient also describes massive neurasthenic complaints from abstinence. He is a handsome, thoroughly masculine, powerful figure. He pines for the fulfilment of his urge and yet, out of a sense of honour, is not yet able to satisfy it. The explanation that this was a congenital and pathological phenomenon had a depressing effect on the one hand and a calming effect on the other. The patient complains that he cannot bring himself to follow his natural instinct, even though he feels that his moral and physical suffering would thereby diminish. His ideal would be to lie down as a man on his lover, to embrace him with all his might and to touch his genitals. He concludes his report with the words:]

May this agonising condition remain far from everyone and may the realisation soon come that it is a congenital pathological one and that those who suffer from it are far more to be pitied than people with serious but nevertheless curable diseases.

8.2 PS3 (1888) Bb 35, 91–3

R: *PS4 (1889) Bb 58, PS5 (1890) Bb 69, PS6 (1891) Bb 82*

I am the eighth child of a craftsman in a small town, who was married three times and knew nothing of contrary sexual feelings, for even in old age he was not averse to the opposite sex. My mother, too, was certainly of a normal disposition; she married early and died of dropsy in her forty-first year. She has a niece, however, of whom I hear that she often meets her sister-in-law in the woods and has conspicuous intercourse with her—I would almost suspect that this cousin of mine is of urning origin.

As a child I was tall, strong and well-fed, so that I was simply called 'the fat one'. I didn't have any childhood illnesses, only acne, which I suffered from for years. Even in later years I was never ill.

The first indication of my infirmity is that as a boy I liked to see or touch a male member. Especially when two men had to sleep together during visits or on journeys, this touching, especially of an erect member, could keep me from sleeping for hours.

Puberty set in before the age of 14, and at the same time, occasionally tempted by others, I also engaged in masturbation, but not frequently and without noticeable harm.

As a grammar school pupil, I was very fond of romantic friendships, and the hugging and kissing of my young friends drew a lot of ridicule. But this love was entirely platonic, not a single erection took place.

In the process, I got into bad company; we boozed, hustled and played all night; I also went out in the evening on the prowl for prostitutes, but I never touched any of them. I was in my twenties when a friend of mine performed coitus with a girl in my presence. Another person wouldn't be able to contain himself with excitement, but I watched the thing with increasing disgust. It was not, however, as I thought at the time, moral repugnance, but physical. Even when I went to a brothel as a student, I could never bring myself to touch such girls, let alone mount them. In the meantime, my physical development continued normally; I came to be 1.78 m tall, had a chest measurement of 96 cm, was well nourished and gave the impression of a strong man.

The only thing feminine about me is that I am very soft and therefore easily moved, sensitive and therefore easily hurt, and I don't smoke. When I was a pupil and smoking was on my list of things to do, prohibition made it attractive to me, but as a student I gave it up immediately because it was too repulsive for me.

For the rest, I may well say of myself that I am intellectually gifted and a very efficient worker; as an educator I may have achieved remarkable things, and, with all goodwill, I am still considered to be very energetic.

When the age of 30 came to an end, my never-satisfied sexual urge caused me so much discomfort that I went to a doctor; my constant erections disturbed my intellectual work, and I sometimes had two pollutions in one night. However, the opposite sex never played a role, but I was always preoccupied with [*LATIN: erect penises*], sometimes also those of stallions and bulls in the same situation.

When the doctor examined my genitals, erection immediately occurred; I was seized with dizziness, fell around the doctor's neck, and there was an outpouring of semen. The doctor laughed and said that all I needed was a woman. I believed it then, too, whereas now I know that the first man who touched me caused this striking process. I followed the doctor's advice and married a well-bred, strong girl, naturally without any inclination, but with the firm intention of being a good husband. I told her that I wanted to have sons, for I was a great lover of children, and so at first, we entered into a marriage of convenience. Love came later for her, but not for me, just as I have never been in love with a female being, neither before nor since.

But I was soon to learn what love was. Nonetheless, with my very strong urge to empty my balls, conjugal visits were very frequent, as a rule three times a day, but I soon fell passionately in love with a younger civil servant whose strength, agility and beauty I could observe at gymnastics. Now I finally realised that my attraction was not to the female but to the male sex, and that I had cheated an excellent woman out of her life's happiness, but certainly without my knowledge and will.

My lover, of course, did not return my affection at all; when I once approached him tenderly while he was lying on the sofa, he pushed me back with kicks, and when, during one of my wife's journeys, I asked him to sleep with me, he went to a prostitute. I played, sang and sighed all night until daylight, when he finally came and laughed at me. After many pleas he came to me more willingly, and when I hugged him, kissed him and brought my member to his, the discharge of semen came quite quickly.

Inwardly, I now fell into a state of misery. From the Bible as well as from classical antiquity, I knew quite well what to think of boy molesters, and it was of little consolation to me that I never touched boys, nor was I even tempted to do so, but only men of about 25 to 30 years of age who were beautifully built and in particular did not smell bad anywhere, for example from the mouth. When I had a man with me in bed or in the bath, I had no regard for propriety or reason, but kissed him from top to bottom, on penis and scrotum, possibly taking both in my mouth, and when the former got an erection or even spilled semen, this was the peak of lustful sensation for me.

Despite all this, I hoped to come to terms with my unnatural impulses with the help of my considerable energy. Despite all reluctance, I still went to my wife, and since she always conceived immediately, she repeatedly gave birth to strong boys, never girls, to whom I was a tender father.

Two things, however, put a stop to my decision: firstly, my wife had a uterine condition which aroused her desire for a man but strictly forbade fertilisation. I therefore first forced myself to get an erection, but then had to interrupt the act before ejaculation. This created an almost insurmountable loathing of the conjugal encounter with my wife, whom, by the way, I manhandled.

In addition, I had to deal with the dread of the female sex in the course of my work. Even the proximity of prostitutes made me feel sick and nauseous, especially the smell of them. But even a handshake with a fine, educated lady made me feel as if I had grasped a toad or a spider.

This quite abnormal condition was later alleviated in a different form. Now, after 16 years of sighing under this misery, the condition is as follows: erections are rare, pollutions have completely disappeared, but the pressure in my scrotum as a result of strong sperm secretion (as the family doctor says) is often so bad that I have to walk with my legs apart. Conjugal intercourse, which my wife demands from time to time, exerts me so much that I tremble and sweat and am exhausted the whole day, whereas intercourse with a man extremely excites, satisfies and makes me mentally and physically fit.

The worst thing is that once sexual excitement has set in, I am absolutely unable to overcome it. My scrotum becomes hard and painful, the facial features become immobile, my eyes are fixed and protrude from their sockets, I tremble with excitement and cannot go out in public in this state. Flows of mucus during urination and defecation increase the unbearable nature of the situation, which I have to put an end to by masturbation if I don't have a friend. But masturbation, just like conjugal intercourse, causes me the deepest tension and dejection.

Help relieve the agonising pressure that weighs on so many unfortunates and drives them to despair.

8.3 PS3 (1888) Bb 36, 93–6

I am 27 years of age; my father was very devoted to sexual pleasure with women, despite or because of his longstanding physical illness. I was brought up by my two sisters. When I was 10-and-a-half years of age, I left my parents' home and went to the grammar school in a neighbouring town. At that time, I was still quite sexually resistant and remained so until my thirteenth year, at which time I unfortunately was led to the vice of masturbation, which I practised to a great extent until my nineteenth year. I first became aware of an inclination towards persons of my own sex at the age of 13, when I suddenly found myself seized by feelings of love for one of my professors, a young, beautiful and blooming man, in whose case my naturally undisclosed and unrequited ardour increased steadily with the years, so that after the fourth year of grammar school (I was 15 years of age at the time), I persuaded my father to send me to another grammar school. My studies were highly successful in the first years; I was praised by my professors as a very talented boy, but due to onanism I gradually noticed a decline in my power of memory, which became particularly noticeable in the VII and VIII classes. Nevertheless, I remained a privileged pupil and graduated with distinction. In Class VI, I felt a deep affection for a very pretty fellow pupil who was years ahead of me, but I soon overcame it. During this time, I also maintained contact with the landlord with whom I lived; this was my first sexual intercourse with another person. This gentleman, although married and the father of several children, at the age of 48, had brought me to this sexual intercourse himself, while I found in the intercourse with him only a mere sexual satisfaction without any aesthetically higher feeling, because he was ugly. I never felt the slightest inclination towards women, although many came my way. During my university years, I twice tried to have relations with pleasure-girls, but never achieved an erection. I am afflicted with the perversion of the sexual instinct.

When I began my university studies, I was overcome by the realisation of the reprehensibility of a passion such as onanism, and I renounced the vice altogether. But I could not come to terms with the strange sexual sensations that plagued me and all the more I tried to banish them. I wrote many letters anonymously to a doctor, but in spite of a lot of money, I received nothing but foolish advice to force myself to have a woman, the result of which I then undertook the attempts mentioned above. I lapsed into complete melancholy, which was puzzling to my family and all my acquaintances. Formerly a cheerful and popular young man, I became asocial, deeply emotionally ill, self-tormenting and suicidal. My great sexual instinct, however, became more and more imperious, and however much I detested myself, I sought and found (not without danger) the possibility of satisfying myself with some strong workers. This intercourse consisted only in lustful groping of the body and the sexual parts, and the copulation of mine with the man's was enough for ejaculation. I have always detested penetrating the anus, although I cannot deny that such desires are not the farthest thing from my mind now; indeed, that despite my otherwise highly idealistic way of thinking and feeling, I would find the greatest pleasure performing this sexual act if I set aside all aesthetic consideration. The ambivalence that I experience in the direction of my sexual instinct is also strange. On the one hand, it is directed towards strong, lusty persons of low status, whose filth and impurity are only a spur for me; this direction grants me the only possibility of ejaculating with lust and pleasure. On the other hand, however, my urge has a purely aesthetic direction towards beautiful urnings, but unfortunately this direction is limited to platonic kisses and embraces, without bringing about a voluptuous excitement whose goal would be the ejection of semen. Despite frequent intercourse with beautiful and fine urnings, I could never bring myself to do so. This unfortunate dichotomy is, in addition to the sadness inherent in the perversion of the desire for sex, another very disastrous one. If I really want to satisfy myself sexually, I have to seek out people of the kind mentioned above and obtaining them is very dangerous. Last year, I had the misfortune of a strong man whom I approached having me arrested: what agonies I had to endure before I experienced the final trial, at which I was acquitted by the benevolence of my judges and the consideration of my official position, although my guilt was clear to everyone. No wonder, that I—unfortunately!—have given myself up to masturbation since then, because other means were lacking. I experience the consequences of this vice, and I have felt them even before that. For eight years I have been shy, terribly nervous and irritable; in society I am sometimes insecure, then again terribly sensitive to everyone, often to unintentional expressions, and unlovable. I know that all this is due to masturbation, and yet I cannot suppress my impulse, the less so because at the time of my striving to conquer it I fell into the neurasthenia you have touched upon, in consequence of which I came to be quite apathetic, so that later I preferred to raise myself up and make myself more lively by moderate masturbation, as it seemed to me. I believe I would revive and come to be a completely different person if I were allowed to satisfy myself according to my urges. But as it is, I suffer terribly from the nervous alterations to which I am exposed, partly through masturbation and partly through abstinence. My attitude to life is very low, I lack the self-confidence and the cheerful appearance of other young people; I suffer from self-tormenting imaginings, and my appearance is therefore a despondent one.

I have certainly also suffered physically. As a boy I had a wonderful soprano voice that enchanted connoisseurs; my musical talent is brilliant. Since puberty, however, I have lost this voice, not only, as is natural, as the high treble voice, but I have completely lost the ability to sing. I only know that I was still able to produce high female tones long after puberty, which asserted itself in my speaking voice; strangely enough, I am still able to do so today, even though these would be beautiful, sonorous chest tones (not deep), which my sense of shame prevents me from allowing to be heard in public. My emotional life is more feminine and soulful. I love music and art passionately and have a great dramatic talent, which I once dreamed of exploiting as an opera singer. By the way, my organ of speech is very sonorous and has come to be described by stage artists as very valuable for the stage in combination with my acting talent. My intellectual capacity is, I believe, not limited, only my memory is very idiosyncratic, and only in relation to things that are interesting to me is it compliant; indeed, here it is astonishingly great. My memory for people in particular is unmistakable. Politics can only arouse little interest in me. I don't love female pursuits—only as a child did I like to occupy myself with such things—and girls were also my companions during my childhood. I forgot to tell you that I have a strong beard (full beard and moustache), on my body there is strong hair growth on my thighs, on my pubic area, little on my chest. My penis is not large, but my testicles are quite big. I believe I have told you the most important features of my nature in these lines.

I am mainly interested in getting a clue about my unpleasant moods. How sad it is to be afflicted with a condition that one must fearfully conceal, and in the concealment of which lies the greatest threat to one's peace of mind.

8.4 PS4 (1889) Bb 61, 131–8

R: *PS5 (1890) Bb 72*

My family is, as far as I know, perfectly healthy sexually. My paternal grandfather died of a lung ailment at the age of 45. He is said to have been a morally perfect character. I can assure the same of my father and mother. I have three younger sisters, unmarried, very talented and popular with everyone because of their excellent and charming character.

We received the most careful education. I completed primary and grammar school. At the age of 17-and-a-half, I was one of the pupils who received the highest test scores for the high school diploma. The principal described me in my report as a person gifted with a fine aesthetic sense and at the same time as having great willpower.

My innermost aspiration from childhood onwards was to become an artist, an actor. Even as a grammar school pupil, I imagined for years that everything I said, did and performed, indeed every movement of my body, every look in my eyes, was acted, and that I was a thoroughly fictitious type. I am filled with ardent enthusiasm for the works of German and classical art; in the perception, recreation and reproduction of any work of art, whether poetic or musical, I am on a par with many a great artist; in the portrayal of tragic moments and passions I can achieve something significant and have a shock effect—I can prove it many times. In the work of art, I really forget everything personal and become a different, freer person. In the realisation of my life's ideal, I failed first because of fierce resistance from my family, then because of a linguistic malady, because of a stammer that I could never completely overcome so that I felt completely secure, and finally because of a lack of psychological and moral stamina, the latter of which is probably due to my sexual relationships. My talent, however, is entirely receptive. That is its barrier. I am practically incapable of producing anything independently, something decent or scientifically significant.

My entire intellectual being consists of a feeling that is perhaps developed to the point of genius (not thinking but feeling). Religiously, despite my Catholic upbringing, I have been a free man since the age of 17, to the regret of my family.

In primary school, when I was six or seven years of age, I socialised with a somewhat older companion who initiated me into sexual secrets. We showed each other our genitals, touched them often, especially on walks, and I still remember that we made the remark that we found other people's touch more pleasant than our own. Erections were still unpleasant for us at that time. Intercourse with this boy did not last long; my friend soon came to dislike me, and from then on, I was always alone in relation to sex. At grammar school and high school, I generally kept my distance from my mates; I was considered an oddball, brooding and somewhat aloof, although everyone was basically well-disposed towards me. I only got to know happy socialising and beer drinking as a student in the fifth semester. When I was 10 or 11 years of age, lying alone in bed, I began to masturbate of my own accord. I don't remember how it happened, but the feeling was intoxicating; I was drunk with childish bliss, and from that day on I practised this vice almost daily for years. Around the same time, I became happily infatuated with a handsome companion; however, I was only able to spend two months in the country with him. That was a short time of first sexual impulses, combined with that sweet longing that can still seize me often enough today. Later, I came into a circle of many children, boys and girls from good society, who came together from the neighbouring houses and played. It was a very large circle, and soon small pairs of lovers were formed, and so I, too, following the example of the others, chose a girl whom I tried to win over and whom I actually succeeded in adoring for a while. I imagined I loved her, and a few times even associated that girl with my erections. At the same time, however, a strong desire arose in me to feel the genitals of my friends as well as my own. This longing has grown ever since; a sense of honour, of shame, kept me from realising the desire. I have never felt a real sexual impulse towards a girl or a woman.

From childhood onwards, I was only interested in figures of my own sex, descriptions of male genitals, as well as pictures and statues. At the age of 15, I developed a deep infatuation for a friend two years older than I, of somewhat stocky build and a rather good-natured face, while at the same time a smaller boy of about 11 or 12 years occupied my imagination. I remember how frightened I was when I once managed to put my hand between his thighs while he was lying unwell in bed, and I was visiting him. It also happened that we hung together on a gymnastic apparatus, and I hugged him very tightly with my legs without him resisting me. Indeed, one day we each lit a small sulphur match, blew it out and handed it to each other without saying a word, as a sign that our love was to be extinguished, and I believe that from then on, we really did have the strength to no longer approach each other in that more violent way which had seemed uncanny and forbidden to us. In the meantime, a real youthful passion for a very intelligent friend of my age and class had taken hold of me at the age of 16. I was blissfully happy when I was able to sit next to him for a whole year; school seemed transfigured to me; our thighs were always intertwined in some way under the bench, and even the slightest touch with this amiable, slender friend aroused the most violent erections in me. I was more passionate than he was, but it did happen from time to time that he, too, seized by sudden madness, pressed me fiercely against him. And it was always his legs, especially his thighs, that excited me with their shape. He wore tight trousers, and I never got tired of looking at his supple growth. I remember that we once sat opposite each other for a whole afternoon and pressed our thighs against each other. At that time, I felt a sharp pain in my testicles afterwards, which I have experienced ever since after every intense, prolonged erection. At the same time, I never dared to give in to my passion completely; every further desire was suppressed to the best of my ability; our relationship remained a friendship—we worked, we very often played music together and we never spoke about sexual things—indeed, I don't remember that we ever kissed each other, no matter how fiercely I longed for it. Only when I was masturbating did I embrace my dear friend in my imagination. This relationship, so happy and unhappy for me, lasted about four years—we had to separate, and in the last days I was stunned with pain. My boyfriend became an officer. We met again a few times later; after a few minutes the old feeling in me had awakened again, but he had become sedate and quiet. Even now we still correspond most cordially. When I was 18 years of age, I heard the word 'onanism' for the first time; I found the explanation in the encyclopaedia, and I, who until then had thoughtlessly and childishly wasted my strength, fell for a while into a state of terrible consternation and self-torment.

Every pollution (accompanied, of course, only by dreams relating to male figures) increased my horror; I imagined consumption, spinal cord diseases, ridiculously even syphilis, and a large part of these thoughts haunt me to this day and embitter my life, for I have not been able to give up on masturbation to this day, despite all my efforts and temporary restrictions. I will only briefly describe my student life. My friends often tried to get me to go out with women, but they never succeeded. In their presence, I sometimes had to embrace a girl; there were even more intrusive scenes from the female side, but I never had even the slightest sexual arousal. Everything was indifferent to me; I was considered a paragon of virtue. I liked to socialise and associate with families and women's society;

I certainly appear there today, where I am very popular. I dance well and a lot if I have to, but I remain completely cold. During my university years I was, on the whole, a happy student. I never had any real idea of my condition. The essence of friendship, as I perceived it, I had worked out in such a way that, from an aesthetic point of view, I could only really love beautiful, slender people. All the friends I really loved appealed to my senses at the same time. I was especially passionately devoted to a truly beautiful journeyman in B. and St. He had, as it were, taken the place of my high-school sweetheart. It happened once in St that he took me to his house at night because I had forgotten my house key; on a second evening, I secretly threw the key into the river myself, and so it happened that I slept together with him twice. The most terrible excitement kept me completely awake, but I did not dare to approach him completely, only at first there were a few light touches; my friend fell asleep, and shame kept me from embracing his beloved body. Those were blissfully sad nights. From that time on, I practised more often the kind of masturbation that I had tried earlier, seduced by a passage in Lessing's *Redemption of Horace*,[1] namely, to undress completely, to take a large mirror from the wall and to look at my whole figure in it. In the absence of a lover, I embraced and kissed my own body, as it were, imagining with desire how much more ardent and intoxicating the real embrace of a lover would have to be. How often, how hotly I wished for a dear bedfellow! Once in B. I thought I was being spoken to by a boy in the night in the manner of a strumpet, and from then on, I often took a lover home with me in my thoughts. And always I did not yet recognise the whole truth of my nature! Once in Berlin, an older, unappealing man, who must have seen through me, pursued me with letters and visits; he wanted to bring me into the company of men. Astonished, contemptuous, I sent him away. I didn't know what he wanted. I always believed that there was perhaps still a great passion for a woman in me, a passion that I, myself, had been able to express so convincingly and strongly in my works of art from an early age—all it would take would be the right woman. I sometimes thought of boy-love, and wished myself transported to the Orient, where boy-love is supposed to be permitted, but it was not until I was 24 that I learned of [*LATIN: anal intercourse*]; I then read articles on pederasty, but it seemed to me that nothing was explained, for I could not possibly place myself in the same line with those 'pederasts' as I found them described; my feeling seemed nobler and at the same time more mysterious.

I now come to the most terrible and exciting period of my life. In the town where I was employed, a deep passion awoke in me for a somewhat older, beautiful and highly talented woman who had been married at the age of 20, but who had been living separately from her husband for many years (not for the world to see, but in the house, for the sake of the children). I had never thought such a thing was possible, although I had been idolised several times by females, for example, by friends of my sisters. I had never believed I could seriously fall in love. It was as if being struck by lightning, and a deep, heartfelt gratitude and love drew me to this woman, who was so like-minded and similar to me in many ways. At the same time, I was intoxicated and thought: This is the love for a woman, in this case you can perhaps give yourself to her. This much is certain: if that woman had been free, if I had found her as an unmarried girl, or if a solution had been possible, I would have made her my bride, my wife, even without the slightest sexual feeling. But in this situation, I tried in the most honest way from the first beginning with all my efforts to the end to transform our relationship into a purely sisterly one, as I felt it to be, but I did not know what I was doing: I had no idea of the great, genuine passion of that woman who, the nobler, the more selfless I appeared to be, the more inflamed she became, until her feeling grew to infinite violence. Let me remain silent about scenes of quiet happiness, of the greatest peace, in which I felt the woman with pride as my own, in which every spiritual impulse, every stirring of tender feeling had an unspoken clarity to us, and then again scenes of the most violent passion on her part, which, in the feeling of my unworthiness, brought me to fits of weeping, to raging expressions, to frenzy, until the woman, frightened, became silent and vowed to do everything and force her heart as I wished. Just think—the relationship lasted four years. Yes, yes, I was guilty, but not as much as it seems. If I had known for certain that I was an urning, if I had had your book in my hands even then, I would have turned away with energy from the beginning; I would have fled the loving woman, instead of seeking her as one in need of being rescued, like from fire, as I will flee every feeling for a female from now on.

O, how often the word was on my lips, how often I wanted to rush to her feet and say: You love a criminal; I do not understand myself, but it is true; I desire only my own sex—push me away, give me the heave, loathe me, but at the same time pity the despicable one. Indeed, how often did I not give her real hints of my condition, but alas, she, who, in spite of her age, in spite of her marriage, was as inexperienced as a child; she did not understand me, and I also believe I would have driven her to death by my frankness. She saw the struggle in me and thought it suppressed passion for her. Even today, after the agonising separation from her, she sees in me her strong hero, her God, and endures life only in the consciousness of my love for her, and now, in truth, it has become my duty to maintain this illusion. Thus, the highest thing there is according to sound human concepts, the full possession of an infinitely loving woman, has been offered to me, and I have had to reject it because of my nature. And during the time of that relationship also came the struggle with my profession, that ever more powerful development of my dramatic talent, my acting—yes, I really did become a viscerally brilliant actor with my gift of empathy—and if I had achieved this goal in reality at that time, I believe that I would also now have been able to bear the abnormality of my nature more easily. During all that time, I passionately desired some of the young people around me, for schoolboys who happened to be doing gymnastics in my garden and with whom I went swimming during the summer. I was happy in the company of my friends whom I knew how to stimulate, artistically, scientifically, humanly, who, since I was one of their own, really revered and loved me. And further—it is pathetic, but true—a young 18-year-old barber's assistant who came to shave me a few times a week: I tried to grab his genitals at that time—and I succeeded!

He sat on my thigh, allowed me to feel him and pressed himself against me during my ejaculation. For the first, for the only time, I held a man's member in my hand, and it was an oppressive pleasure to feel and see his erection. It happened five or six times, then my willpower won out—the journeyman came to me for many more weeks, but I conquered myself and just let him come and go. In the one case the noblest, best woman who awaited me with ardent enthusiasm, in the other case a journeyman barber whose genitals I touched in the meantime! You can imagine my reproaches, my disruption, my almost insane state. Even today, knowing my nature, I consider that affair dishonourable, mean and wretched. But I could not, I cannot be faithful to a woman, whereas now I know I can be faithful to a lover, even if I do not possess him.

Listen to the conclusion of my confession! I arrived in T.; my condition has remained the same. But for a year now, I have found a lover who possesses my whole heart, my life. The sweetest, most longing infatuation, the most selfless love and the hottest sexual passion chain me to this boy. He is a 16-year-old high school student, the son of a family we are friends with. I try to bring him up, encourage him, work with him (he is not the best at school). I help him with his studies, go to his teachers when it is necessary, and I try to teach him diligence and energise him in every way. I give him as much pleasure as I can—I want him to become a capable, happy person.

And that's the reason why I don't fully embrace him; I don't want to harm him psychologically and morally; he loves me and I could possess him if I wanted to. He is strongly developed, intelligent, fierce and tender at the same time. The other day he said, 'O why can't you and I marry each other?' He has three brothers, but I am dearest to his heart—the brother and friend with whom he wants to be day and night! A few times we happened to sleep together, but I always clenched my teeth and mustered all my strength so as not to sink into the stream of happiness, even to be able to reject the dear fellow—that's how it is with me now, and this love lasts: I am not unfaithful to it; other companions hardly tempt me. I feel completely as a man and have always felt only as a man, despite my receptive spirit. My greatest happiness would be to lie naked in bed with my beloved, to enclose him tightly with arms and legs and to imitate coitus. His head would have to lie on my chest and my face buried in his dear woollen head. If I could enjoy this happiness for only one night, I would no longer be completely unhappy, for I would then know that the highest sensual pleasure of life had once been granted to me, and in the memory of it I could, as I believe, continue to bear life alone, as a widower. The calm, lasting physical and spiritual possession of the beloved, for whom I could endure the bitterest pains, the worst adversities, for whom I could die at any moment, would make me the most blessed person in the world, a true man who would fulfil his daily life's work with joy and perseverance. That is my firm conviction. I have no desire to have a family of my own.

Finally, it remains for me to describe myself physically. I am tall and lean of strong bone structure, but not very strong. My legs are long and somewhat fuller than my upper body and arms. I am a good walker, swimmer and skater. My sexual parts are, I believe, quite normal, my testicles at times hanging down (a consequence of onanism?), then again firmly attached, even in a resting state. My penis is long and stiff during erection. My health is quite good, my body tough in bearing heat and cold. Apart from diphtheria, I have not yet suffered any serious illness. My face is sharply marked, and my light-coloured hair growth is luxuriant.

I have long since renounced masturbation. However, if I wake up at night and am very excited, or if my sexual excitement cannot be overcome in the morning or evening, I firmly imagine that I am lying next to my lover, I wrap my arms around my own body, put the blanket between my thighs, and imitate coitus until ejaculation occurs in an instant. On average, this happens every 8 to 14 days. I often have to fight it for longer, and I often have to give in to the sexual urge for several days in a row. Pollutions are not quite regular, often several nights in a row, then they stop again for three or four weeks. So far, I have been quite spared nervous pains, but sometimes I feel very miserable and dull, feel pressure in my head, pains in my back, a pulling in my legs, but so far these conditions have always passed.

My family, even the family doctor, believes that the little nervousness is the result of my profession, my diligence. The whole world thinks I am a thoroughly honourable, solid, even particularly strict, moral young man.

No one suspects my true nature, only you, a stranger, you alone know me now, and in fact more precisely than my father and mother, any friend, woman, or lover. It has been a blessing to me to be allowed to reveal the oppressive secret of my own nature for once.

8.5 PS5 (1890) Bb 63, 113–7

R: *PS6 (1891) Bb 78*

Your writing, *Die conträre Sexualempfindung vor dem Forum* (Contrary sexual feeling before the forum),[2] which I have just put down, has aroused my interest to a high degree. It is, however, only a weak attempt to make the abnormal phenomenon—which occurs more frequently than you suspect—comprehensible to wider circles and to prove that the exercise of the natural instinct, even if in a form other than the conventional one, cannot possibly be punishable.

If truly wise men were to create the laws, they would have to say to themselves that people cannot be punished for inclinations which nature has placed in them. Is there any creature more pitiful than a man who, endowed with many virtues of mind and heart, one day makes the dreadful discovery that he is sexually different from other men? In all ways, he finds stones of offence: in social intercourse with the opposite sex, he is an insensitive being who, by his reserve, arouses the astonishment and ridicule of men and, by his restraint, arouses desires in sensual women which he is incapable of satisfying. There is no unalloyed pleasure for him anywhere, for almost all phenomena of social, literary and artistic life are based on the sensual intercourse of the two sexes. The most ideal poems deal with their love affair, and where others find exaltation, it arouses in the urning bitterness and deep sorrow of soul over the undeserved fate. He cannot even come to terms with his parents and brothers and sisters: there is always something strange between them; they do not know how to explain his changing moods, and when he returns home from society exhausted by the annoying compulsion of pretence—he is not allowed to present himself as he is—they consider him capricious and hypochondriacal. And this creature, abused by nature, should be punished when the exuberant feeling runs riot in the arms of a like-minded person?

One does not regard the urning as a lowly being, that would be erroneous. He may be the most perfect creation of nature. I know some whose disposition is so noble that I have never observed it in normal people. Receptive to the arts in the most ideal direction, the urning usually also raves about the beauties of nature; he loves the world of flowers and plants, which, in their sexless beauty, give him almost the only unadulterated pleasure. He loves people and has compassion for their faults and weaknesses, because he knows from his own sad experience how powerful the innate instinct in man is, whether for good or evil. In many cases, he combines masculine strength and willpower with the tenderness of feminine feeling, and if—as often happens—he is also beautiful in form, he really is nature's model creation in his overall characteristics.

I was attracted to men during my childhood and suffered a lot from this inclination. For as a straight, open character, every lie repelled me and yet I lied for as long as I could remember. No one was allowed to suspect what I felt. My awe of the law was so strong that even in secret, I was incapable of any action that would persecute it. That is why I avoided intercourse with other urnings and sought satisfaction of the sexual urge in masturbation. I used to think that my unhappy inclination was due to a pathological state of mind, so I turned to Professor L. in W. I must have inspired a lot of pity in him, but he could not help me. Nevertheless, I left him reassured; my heart had been lightened by the information, and I gained the courage to do what my nature urged me to do. The professor had advised me to live in the countryside for a while to strengthen my nerves, but I tried to numb myself by socialising with my peers. At that time, I had the opportunity to socialise with a whole group of like-minded people who, however, did not instil any deeper interest in me; the sensual intercourse with them filled me afterwards with deep regret, and when I did not encounter the same feelings where heartfelt affection drew me, I returned home more nervous, irritable and unhappy than ever.

I am now in my thirty-third year. A sick soul lives in a body that is almost 6 feet high and strangely bristles with health. The constant compulsion and pretence, which are prescribed to me by prejudice, destroy my spirit and corrupt my soul. Formerly the idol of my mother, I must now accuse myself of gradual brutalisation, and yet I used to be regarded as a model of fine tact and the most delicate refinement. I wish to die, but as long as my poor mother lives, I must not kill myself. What good is life to me? A miserable youth is followed by a joyless old age. The urning must die young, for all the joys of old age, as they come to him through children and grandchildren, are denied him, and he is left with nothing but the agonising consciousness of a life missed through no fault of his own. Thousands find themselves in this terrible situation. Should not everything come to the rescue of these thousands from the oppressive feeling that they have a secret to hide, the discovery of which ranks them well below the criminal?

This secret has a paralysing effect on every spiritual and mental impulse and causes the wasting away of great talents; the result, however, is madness and suicide. If it is in your power to protect these unfortunates from public opinion, do it. You will save many noble people and among them ingenious natures from ruin.

Before I close these lines, I would like to share with you a thought that has occupied my mind a great deal recently. Perhaps there is a way to heal through suggestion. There is so much talk about the scientific use of magnetism; would it not be possible to cure the disease by a magnetic cure? I would gladly put myself at your disposal, and if I succeeded—I don't even dare to hope—it would be a triumph beyond compare.

8.6 NF (1891) Bb 1, 97–102

R: PS7 (1892) Bb 137, PS8 (1893) Bb 137

I was born out of wedlock in 1858. Only late in life, following the dark traces of my origins, did I gain knowledge about the person of my parents. Unfortunately, this information is very scanty and incomplete. Father and mother were cousins. Father died three years ago, later married elsewhere, and fathered several—as far as I know—healthy children.

I don't believe that my father had contrary sexual feelings. I saw him several times as a child, without knowing that he was my father. He was a strong male figure. Incidentally, he was said to have been sexually ill at the time of my birth or earlier.

I saw my mother several times on the street but did not know at the time that she was my mother. My mother was probably about 24 years of age when I was born. She was of tall stature, swift, energetic movements and determined character. At the time of my birth, she was said to have travelled a lot in men's clothing, wore her hair short, smoked a long pipe and was generally conspicuous for her eccentric nature. She had an excellent education, is said to have been beautiful in her youth, left behind a fortune that is very significant by today's standards, but died unmarried.

From all of this, one would come to the conclusion that she was homosexually inclined or had some abnormalities. On the other hand, my mother gave birth to a girl several years before I was born. This stepsister, unknown to me personally, married young, but poisoned herself in the first years of the marriage for reasons unknown to me.

I am 1.70 m tall, 92 cm in the waist and 102 cm around the hips, so I think I have a somewhat strongly developed pelvis. My fat padding has always been well developed. Bone structure strong. Musculature well developed, but perhaps due to lack of exercise, perhaps under the influence of early and constantly strong masturbation, not quite developed, so that I appear stronger than I am. Hair on head and beard normal. Hair on genitals somewhat sparse. The rest of my body is almost hairless. The rest of my appearance is quite masculine. Gait, bearing, voice are those of an adult man, and other urnings have often told me that they never saw my passion. I have served in the military and have always enjoyed all the knightly exercises—riding, fencing, swimming and so on.

My first education came to me through a clergyman. I had few actual playmates. The family life of my foster parents was irreproachable. In October 1861 I was sent to an institute. It was there that I committed my first perverted acts, which I will come to in more detail in the description of the development of my sexual life.

I graduated from grammar school, served my voluntary year, then studied forestry and am now an estate manager. In the first years of my life, my intellectual development was very slow. I did not learn to speak until my third year, which gave further credence to the assumption that I had hydrocephalus. From school onwards, my mental development was normal, I even learned easily, but I was never able to concentrate my activities on one particular point. I have a great sense for art and aesthetics, but almost no sense at all for music. My character was the worst imaginable in earlier years. Without being able to give a reason for it, a complete change has taken place within the last 12 years. Today I hate nothing more than lying and no longer tell untruths, even in jest. In money matters, without being stingy, I have become a good steward.

Enough that today, I look back on past times with deep shame and, if I could be freed from my unfortunate sexual perversion or perversity, would rightly consider myself a consummate gentleman. I am good-natured, always ready to do good within the bounds of my means, usually of a cheerful character, a welcome companion. I have no trace of the nervous irritability so often emphasised in fellow sufferers. Nor do I lack personal courage. In the first stages of my development, there is nothing to suggest an abnormality. Even as a child, I liked to lie on my stomach in bed and often slid voluptuously back and forth on my stomach in the morning, which my foster parents often laughed about. But I don't remember ever having had any feelings of desire. I never particularly sought girls as playmates, nor did I ever play with dolls. I heard talk of sexual things early on. But I never thought anything of it. Even in my dream life, sexuality did not come up at that time. Nor in my dealings with boys of the same age. I believe I may claim that my sexual life only awakened after I had been seduced into mutual masturbation by a room-mate in my thirteenth year at the institute. Ejaculation did not take place at that time, only about a year later. Nevertheless, I gave myself up to the vice of masturbation with full passion. At that time, however, the first signs of homosexual inclination appeared. Young, strong men, market workers, labourers and soldiers all entered my dream life and played a major role in my masturbatory fantasies. The first inclination towards pederasty, especially passive sodomy, was already apparent. Up to the age of 14, I very often made mutual attempts at sodomy with my seducer, but we never succeeded in achieving [*LATIN: penetration*]. At the same time, I still had a weak inclination towards the female sex. About half a year after my first onanism, I was once with a prostitute, but I had neither ejaculation nor any particular feeling of desire. Later, until I was 19, I had intercourse in brothels about six times. Erection and ejaculation occurred promptly, but without an outstanding feeling of desire. Masturbation, especially mutual, was at least as dear to me. I never had a 'grammar school love affair'. About 10 years ago, when I was at the baths of H., I believed that love awoke in me for a strikingly beautiful lady from a highly respected family. I felt comfortable in her proximity and thought myself happy when I found reciprocal love. This relationship also kept me from masturbation for a while, but I was afraid that I would not be able to fulfil my marital duties, weakened by many years of masturbation. When we came to a physical separation, the feeling cooled very quickly; I realised that I had deceived myself, and after about two years I was able to learn without jealousy that the young lady had married. My inclination towards women—if I ever possessed such a thing at all—cooled more and more. Two-and-a-half years ago, when I visited a brothel in H. with very virile friends, I had my last sexual intercourse. An erection still took place, an ejaculation no longer. Women have come to mean nothing to me; the prostitute who behaves insolently arouses my displeasure. I like to converse with witty women, especially older ones, although I am often clumsy and awkward, even tactless, in their company. I have never been able to find any charm in the bodily forms of women.

But back to the perverse direction. When I came to H. at the age of 14, I lost contact with my lover and seducer. He was a few years older than I and had become a civil servant. As such, I met him again on a train when I was 19. We interrupted the journey by necessity, slept together and tried to sodomise each other, but the pain prevented us from achieving [*LATIN: penetration*]. We contented ourselves with mutual masturbation. In H. I had sexual intercourse with two fellow pupils, but this intercourse was limited to very frequent mutual masturbation, as they were not inclined to pederasty. In the last year of my stay (at 19 years of age), I had intercourse with a third, also masturbating, but our intercourse was more intimate, and we always undressed and engaged in mutual masturbation in bed. From Easter 1869 to July 1870, I had no lover. I masturbated alone. At the outbreak of the war, I volunteered, but without being accepted. A former schoolmate, who had developed into a strikingly beautiful person, surrendered to me. I was forced to spend a night with him in a miserable hotel with one bed. Although we had not had sexual intercourse as pupils, he was inclined towards my courtship and attempted sodomy. Here, too, it did not succeed because of the pain, but [*LATIN: ejaculation onto my anus*] occurred during the attempts. Even today, I remember the previously undreamed-of feeling of lust. I met this friend several times after the war, but later our intercourse was limited to masturbation.

During the following 18 years or so, I only had the opportunity to have homosexual intercourse twice. First, in the winter of 1879, I met a handsome hussar in a railway coach. I persuaded him to sleep with me at an inn. Later, he confessed to me that he had already mutually masturbated with the son of a landowner from his town. I could not persuade him to become a pederast. On the other hand, I caused him to ejaculate by [*LATIN: receiving his penis in my mouth*]. This method did not give me satisfaction, but disgust. I never practised it again later, nor did I ever allow [*LATIN: my penis being received in another's mouth*]. In 1887 I made the acquaintance of a sailor, also on a train, and induced him to stay with me at a hotel. Although he said he had never practised sodomy, he immediately showed himself willing to do so, was obviously very sensually aroused, immediately had erections and performed the act with obvious passion. It was the first time that sodomy had succeeded. I had terrible pain, but also infinite pleasure.

My sexual life has undergone a radical change during my stay here. I have found how easy it is to find people here, partly for money, partly out of inclination, who respond to our inclinations. I have not been spared any dismal experiences with criminals. Until the end of last year, since then I have only masturbated mutually for fear of being venereally ill, and I have savoured the pleasure of male love, especially in the sense of passive sodomy. I have never actively sodomised, if only because I could not find anyone who could stand the pain.

I look for my lovers mainly among the cavalry, the sailors and possibly the workers, especially butchers and blacksmiths. I am particularly attracted to robust builds with a healthy complexion. Leather commissary breeches have their own attraction for me. I have no preference for kissing or flirting. I also love big, hard and well-worked hands.

I do not want it to go unmentioned that I have great self-control under certain circumstances.

As an estate manager, I inhabited a large house. My personal servant was a beautiful young man who had served in the hussars. After I had once spoken to him in general about the matter and learned that he was unapproachable, I lived closely with the young man for years, enjoyed his beauty, but never touched him. I believe that he still knows nothing of my passion.

Similarly, two-and-a-half years ago in C. I made the acquaintance of a sailor whom my friends and I regard as the most beautiful man we know. After an absence of more than two years, he accepted an invitation to visit me a few weeks ago. I arranged it so that we slept in the same room, and I burned with desire to get closer to him. Before that, however, I investigated him in private, and when I learned that he despised everything that had to do with male love, I could not bring myself to approach him any further. We slept in the same room for weeks. I always enjoyed his beautiful body (in the first few days I was even sexually aroused), and I took Roman baths with him to see his beautiful body naked—but he never found out about my passion. Even today, I have an ideal, platonic relationship with the young man, who, by the way, possesses an education and a beautiful gift for poetry that is rare for his class.

I did not have any clarity about my condition until I was 38.[3] I always believed that I had only been weaned from womanhood through early and intensively continued masturbation, and I always hoped that once 'the right' girl came along, I would be able to give up masturbation and find pleasure in womanhood. I fully recognised my condition only after I had made the acquaintance of my fellow sufferers and companions. At first, I was horrified, but later I came to terms with my fate as something not of my own making. I also made no further attempts to resist the temptation.

About two or three weeks ago, *Psychopathia Sexualis* fell into my hands. This work made an unexpectedly deep impression. At first, I read the work with undoubtedly lascivious interest. The description of the sexual congress of the mujerados,[4] for example, excited me immensely. The thought that a young, strong man would come to be emasculated in this way in order to later serve a whole tribe of wild, strong and sensual Indians passively was so arousing that I masturbated five times in the next two days, dreaming of myself as such a presumptive mujerado. However, the further I progressed in reading the work, the more the moral seriousness of it became clear to me, the more I felt disgust at my present situation, the clearer it became to me that I must do everything to bring about a change in my present condition, if at all possible. When I had read through the work, I made up my mind to seek help from the author.

The reading of the aforementioned work has undoubtedly been successful. Since then, I have only masturbated twice and only twice with cavalrymen. In all cases, I have had considerably less pleasure and satisfaction than before, and always have the feeling, 'Oh, if only you could stop doing that!' Nevertheless, I confess that even now, I immediately get erections when dealing with beautiful soldiers.

Finally, I would like to add that despite or perhaps because of my frequent masturbation, I have never had pollutions. The discharge of semen, which, by the way, usually consists of only a few drops and has always done so, only occurs after prolonged friction. If for some reason I have not masturbated for a long time, the semen is ejaculated more quickly and abundantly. Hansen tried in vain to hypnotise me about 12 years ago.[5]

8.7 NF (1891) BB 11, 123–7

R: *PS7 (1892) Bb 121, PS8 (1893) Bb 121*

In order to give my unfortunate state of illness the right name, I will say from the outset that it has all the characteristics that you call *effeminatio* in your work *Psychopathia Sexualis.*

I am now 38 years of age and, thanks to my abnormality, have lived a life so full of nameless agony that I am often amazed at the power of suffering that is given to man. Lately, the consciousness of the suffering I have overcome has instilled in me a kind of self-respect that alone can make life somewhat bearable for me.

But I will now endeavour to give a true account of my condition. I am physically healthy, have never, as far as I can remember, suffered any serious illness and come from a healthy family. Admittedly, my parents, both of them, are very excitable natures, my father of a so-called choleric, my mother of a sanguine temperament with a strong tendency to gloomy melancholy. She is an extremely lively woman, popular for her kindness and active help, but with a strong need for affection and a lack of self-confidence. All these qualities were also pronounced in her father. I emphasise this fact because I am said to emulate these two people, and as far as the latter two qualities are concerned, I can see the resemblance myself. I have always believed that my love for my own sex was a consequence of these qualities. But even if I made attempts to break the bond that magically draws me to the man by strengthening myself, by pretending to be capable, there is still a residue that I cannot drive out of my blood. As far as my memories carry me, everywhere I see this enigmatic, elemental longing for a lover. Admittedly, its very first expression was of a crude nature. I don't remember whether I was already 10 years old when I suddenly found myself lying in bed in broad daylight, pressing on my genitals to evoke new, intoxicating feelings, imagining strong sensual manipulations by a man in my surroundings. Only many years later did I learn that this was masturbation. In the early days I was so frightened and so darkened by the mysteriousness of my urge that I made my first suicide attempt at that time. If only I had carried it out! For what followed was a series of such violent shocks of soul and body that they wrapped themselves around my heart like a chain, narrowed it, made it hard and raw. To say it right here, to this day masturbation has not let me out of its claws, it has resisted all attempts, all efforts, and has almost completely broken my desire to resist it. Three or four times I have left it altogether for months, mostly under the influence of mental agitation.

At the age of about 13 I had my first love. Today, I remember that my greatest desire at that time was to kiss the fresh red lips of my schoolmate. It was a longing filled with romantic dreams. It came to a head at the age of 15 or 16, when I suffered for the first time the maddening torment of jealousy, which is more consuming than natural love can be. This second period of love lasted for years, although I was with the object of my love for only a few days, and then we did not see each other again for 15 years. Little by little, my feelings cooled, and then I fell madly in love several more times with other men who, in all but one case, were my peers.

My love—please allow me to use this expression for a feeling condemned by most of humanity—has never been returned. I have never interacted with a man in a way that should shun the light of day, and no one has ever had more than an ordinary interest in me, although one of my idolised friends has guessed my secret desire. And yet I have consumed myself in ardent longing for manly love. In my opinion, my feelings in this regard are entirely those of a loving woman, and I notice with horror that my sensual ideas resemble those of a woman more and more. During the periods in which I am free from a certain love, my desire degenerates to the extent that I conjure up very coarse sensual ideas in my masturbatory manipulations. But I can still fight against this in the end. However, every attempt to suppress love is in vain. For a year now, I have again been suffering from such an exuberance of feeling and have pondered so much over its idiosyncrasies that I believe I can describe my feelings faithfully.

My interest always comes to me through physical beauty. I have made the peculiar observation that I have never loved a bearded man. This leads to the assumption that I am in love with a so-called boy, that I am paying homage to so-called boy-love. That is not correct. For on closer contact, this sensual attraction is joined by an interest in the intellect. And this opens the round of torments. I become seized by such a deep inclination that I connect with a kind of willingness to sacrifice. Trust is gained in me, and such a warm friendship could arise from this reciprocity if the demon did not slumber at the bottom of my soul, urging me to the most intimate union, which is only permitted between people of different sexes. My whole being longs for it, every fibre twitches for it, and in hot, glowing passion I consume myself. I am astonished that I am able to express feelings here in so few words, feelings that have burrowed through my whole being. Admittedly, I have had to learn through years of struggle to conceal my inclination, to smile where I came to be torn by pain. For since I never found love in return, I have only known the torments of love. Jealousy, insane, mind-darkening jealousy of anyone and everyone to whom the one I secretly loved even cast a friendly glance.

I have emphasised the mental moment in order to show how deeply ingrained my abnormal inclination is. Never have I felt even a hint of sensual love for the opposite sex. The idea of having to have sensual intercourse with the opposite sex is repugnant to me. Several times I have suffered enough from being assured of the love of young girls. Like any young man, I have enjoyed modern social pleasures, including dancing. It gives me pleasure to dance, but I would only be happy if I could dance with men as a girl.

I would like to emphasise once again that my love is thoroughly sensual. How else could I explain that the touch of a lover's hand, often the mere sight of him, gives me heart palpitations and erections! I have used all the means at my disposal to tear this 'love' out of my—let us say 'heart'. I have tried to numb it through masturbation, to drag it into the mud so that I can rise above it. (About 10 years ago, during such a love epoch, I detested masturbation and felt as if my love feeling ennobled me.) I still have the delusion that if my lover told me that he loved me reciprocally, that he loved 'only me', I would gladly do without sensual satisfaction and rest in his faithful arms. But that is certainly self-deception.

Honourable Sir! I have a responsible profession, and I believe I can assure you that my abnormal tendency will never come to remove me, even by a hair's breadth, from the duty I must perform. I am not mad, except for this abnormality, and I could be content, after all. But I have suffered too much, especially in the last year, not to look forward with horror to the future, which will certainly not bring me the fulfilment of the wish that continues to glow under the ashes, namely, to possess a lover who understands me and reciprocates my love. Such a relationship alone would truly make me inwardly happy. I have thought a lot about the origin of my abnormality, especially because I believe I must assume that it is not inherited. I believe that masturbation has inflamed the innate feeling to blazing embers. I could have put an end to the whole misery long ago, since I have no fear of death at all and find no warning against suicide in religion, which, strangely enough, has not withdrawn from my impure heart. But the awareness that I am not the only one to blame for the fact that a worm has gnawed away at my whole life from the bud onwards and a certain vitality that has just recently sprouted from unspeakable grief lead me to dare to try for a modest happiness in life that might be built up on a completely new basis after all. Something that fills the heart. I believe that I could be happy under the influence of quiet family life. But I must not conceal from you that the thought of a conjugal life with a woman is dreadful to me and that I would undertake this whole attempt to turn my life around with a bleeding heart, because in doing so I would radically break with the hope that is still alive, namely, with the delusion that fate could still bring me the happiness I have dreamed of. This delusion is so deeply ingrained in me that I fear only hypnotic suggestion can help me.

If you can give me some advice, you would make me infinitely happy. Your most urgent advice will probably bring about the cessation of masturbation. How gladly I would follow it! But if I do not have direct physical, perhaps mechanical means at hand, I will probably not be able to tear myself away from this vice. All the less so because I fear that my nature has become accustomed to it through years of practice. Of course, I have not been spared the consequences, even if they are not as gruesome as they are often described. I suffer from slight nervousness, am weakened and suffer periodically from indigestion, but I can still stand the strain quite well and, if it is not too great, take pleasure in it. I am gloomy but can be quite cheerful and fortunately enjoy my profession and have an interest in many things, especially music, art and fiction. I have never enjoyed feminine pursuits.

As you can imagine from the above, I like to be with men, especially beautiful ones, but I have never entered into comfortable relationships with them. A wide gulf separates me from them.

Addendum. I fear that I have not described my sexual life precisely enough in the foregoing. It consists only in masturbation, but I allow myself to be influenced by almost all the abominable ideas that come to be called [*LATIN: inter-femoral sex, ejaculation in the mouth*] and so on.

My role in this is passive. These ideas change and pass completely over into the desire of mating when a passion puts me under its spell. The fight against such a passion is terrible because my soul is also involved. I long for the closest, most perfect union conceivable between two people, constant togetherness, common interests, unlimited trust, sexual union. I think to myself that natural love differs from this only in the degree of warmth that remains below the boiling point of our passion. Right now, I am fighting that battle again, violently choking down the insane passion that has held me captive for so long now. For nights I toss and turn, haunted by the image of the one for whose love I would give all I have.

How deeply sad it is that the noblest thing that has come to man, friendship, is prevented by mean sensual feelings!

Once again, I would like to emphasise that I cannot decide to change my sex life through sexual intercourse with the opposite sex. The idea of such intercourse is disgusting to me.

Notes

1. Gotthold Ephraim Lessing (1729–1781) was a German novelist and philosopher who published *Die Rettungen des Horaz* in 1754.
2. Richard von Krafft-Ebing, 'Die conträre Sexualempfindung vor dem Forum', *Jarbücher für Psychiatrie* 6 (1885): 34–47.
3. Some uncertainty over age since author says at the start that he was born in 1858, which would make him thirty-three at the time of writing.
4. 'Mujerados' were men magically transformed into women for passive sexual purposes. Krafft-Ebing included a short description of this in each edition from 1888 onwards.
5. Carl Hansen (1833–1897) was a Danish 'magnetist' and stage hypnotist.

CHAPTER 9

Psychic Hermaphrodites

9.1 PS5 (1890) Bb 62, 110–3

R: *PS6 (1891) Bb 77, PS7 (1892) Bb 108, PS8 (1893) Bb 108, PS9 (1894) Bb 107*

According to my ancestry, I am rather heavily burdened. My paternal grandfather was a lively bon vivant and speculator, my father a man of good character, but he has been suffering from *folie circulaire* (manic depression) for more than 30 years without being seriously hindered in his profession. My mother, like her father, suffers from stenocardial seizures. My mother's father and brother are said to have been sexually hyperaesthetic. My only sister, older by nine years, was twice subjected to eclamptic seizures, was religiously exalted in the pubertal years, probably also sexually hyperaesthetic. She struggled for years with severe hysterical neurosis (but is now completely healthy).

As a late-born only son, I was the apple of my mother's eye, and it is only thanks to her tireless care that I recovered completely as a youngster, after having suffered all kinds of childhood illnesses as a child and a boy (hydrocephalus, morbilli, croup, variola, and at 18 years of age, a year of chronic intestinal catarrh). My mother, who was strictly religious, brought me up in this way, without making me angry, and imprinted on me as the highest moral principle an unbending sense of duty, which was developed

D. Pretsell, *Queer Voices in the Works of Richard von Krafft-Ebing, 1883–1901*, Genders and Sexualities in History,
https://doi.org/10.1007/978-3-031-17331-8_9

to the point of brusqueness by a teacher whom I still call friend. Since I spent the greater part of my childhood in bed due to my sickliness, I was dependent on quiet activities, especially reading, and thus came to be a boy who was not blasé, but precocious. Even between the age of eight and nine, I was most interested in the passages in books about injuries or operations that beautiful girls or women had to undergo. For example, a story about a girl getting a thorn in her foot and having it removed by a boy caused me great excitement; indeed, I had an erection every time I looked at the relevant, not at all lascivious picture. As often as possible, I watched chickens being stabbed, and if I missed the sight, I at least looked at the traces of blood with lustful horror and stroked the still warm bodies of the animals. I must emphasise that I have always been a great lover of animals and that the slaughter of larger animals, even the vivisection of frogs, filled me with disgust and pity.

Even today, the stabbing of chickens has a great sexual attraction for me, especially the holding of them, which gives me palpitations and precordial pressure. It is interesting that my dad has a passion for tying the hands of girls and young women. As I believe, another of my sexual abnormalities is also due to this cruel streak in me. As I will describe in more detail later, one of my favourite games was improvised puppet theatre, in which I gave the material to the participants. There was almost always a young girl who had to undergo a painful operation on her foot on the strict orders of her father, whom I portrayed. The more the girl-doll wailed, the higher my satisfaction rose. The reason why I chose the foot as a constant surgical field is as follows: as a little boy I happened to be there when my older sister was changing her stockings. When she quickly hid her feet, it caught my attention, and soon the sight of her bare feet up to her ankles became the ideal of my longing. Of course, this only served to make my sister even more cautious, and so an eternal battle developed, during which on my part I employed all the weapons of cunning and flattery up to explosions of anger until my seventeenth year. Otherwise, I was highly indifferent to my sister; her foot is even repugnant to me. For lack of something better, I also made do with the feet of maids; male feet left me cold. My most longing wish would have been to be allowed to cut the nails or, pardon my French, the corns on a beautiful female foot. My lustful dreams revolved around these things, and I actually turned to the study of medicine in the expectation of finding an opportunity to satisfy my desires or to cure them. Thank God that the latter succeeded. After I had made the first dissection of a female lower limb, the unfortunate spell left me; I say unfortunate because I was always deeply ashamed of myself for having these urges. I think I can spare myself further details, since this strange infatuation, which even inspired me to write poems, has already been portrayed several times.

Now to the last page of my sexual aberrations.

I was about 13 years of age and just beginning to mature when a schoolmate who was temporarily staying with us teased me once in the evening by poking at me with his bare foot from under the covers. I caught his foot and immediately became highly excited, which was followed by a pollution, the first I had ever had. The boy was conspicuously girlish in build and also mentally so. Another companion with very small and delicate hands and feet, whom I once saw in the bath, also excited me immensely. I sometimes thought it a great happiness to be able to lie in bed with one of them, but closer sexual intercourse that went beyond an embrace did not even occur to me. Incidentally, I always rejected such thoughts with disgust. A few years later, between the ages of 16 and 18, I met two boys who awakened my sexual feelings. When I fooled around with them, I immediately had erections. Both were very energetic, fresh, but delicately built boys of childlike appearance. With the onset of puberty, I lost all interest in each of them, even though I retained a warm, friendly affection for both of them. I would never have let myself be tempted into lewd acts with them.

When I entered university, I completely forgot about these aberrations of my [*LATIN: sexual desire*], but out of principle I refrained from any sexual intercourse until I was 24, despite the scorn of my colleagues. When the pollutions became too frequent and I had to fear that I might acquire cerebral asthenia[1] [*LATIN: from abstinence*], I threw myself into the arms of normal sexual life, and to be sure, although I enjoy it rather emphatically, for my greatest good.

The fact that I am almost impotent towards [*LATIN: prostitutes*], that the naked body of a woman disgusts rather than excites me, is probably connected with the special subjects in which I was active for years.

The nude always satisfies me most when I can hold on to the idea of a girl; but since, on the other hand, the idea of the girl coming to be satisfied by someone else besides myself is unbearable to me, I have for years found it absolutely necessary for my mental equilibrium to indulge myself in a kept woman, despite the oppressive pecuniary sacrifices, and only a virgin. Otherwise, the silliest jealousy makes me completely incapable of work. I must also mention that I was platonically in love for the first time when I was 13 years of age, and since then I have often pined away in love. What should distinguish my case above all others is that I have not once in my life masturbated.

A few weeks ago, I was frightened by a sleep in which I dreamt of a [*LATIN: naked boy*] and from which I awoke with an erection.

Finally, I dare to take on the unpleasant task of outlining my [*LATIN: present status*]. Of medium height, of slightly built frame, skull dolichocephalic with a dent in the occipital scales, 59 cm circumference, frontal humps strongly protruding, somewhat neuropathic gaze. Pupils moderately dilated, dentition very defective. Musculature strong, tight. Strong hair growth, blond. Varicocele on the left; a too short frenulum, which prevented me from coitus—I cut myself three years ago. Since then, ejaculation retarded, sensation of lust considerably diminished.

Choleric temperament, quick perception, good talent for association, energetic, very persistent for a hereditarian, learn languages easily, have a good ear, otherwise no talent for the fine arts. Dutiful, but always filled with [*LATIN: tiredness of life*]; prevented from committing suicide only by my religion and consideration for my adored mother. Otherwise, a typical suicide candidate. Ambitious, jealous, paralysophobic, left-handed. Tainted by socialist ideas. Addicted to adventure, courageous—decided never to marry.

9.2 NF (1890) Bb 1, 39–43

I am in my thirty-first year, the first-born among four brothers and also have five living sisters. The health of my family is very good. My father died at the age of 42 from a severe throat complaint. I don't really know the health condition of my paternal grandparents; I only know that they both died when they were about 50–60 years of age. My mother's parents were very healthy. Grandfather died in his seventieth year, grandmother in her eighty-second year from pneumonia. As far back as I can remember in my childhood years, as a boy of eight, I imagined it a great pleasure to be martyred while naked and then hung by my genitals.

Even as a child of five to six, a feeling of love stirred in me, the object of which was a girl of the same age. We always looked for a place where we were undisturbed, covered ourselves either with a cloth or with an umbrella and kissed to our hearts' content. I came to masturbation partly through myself and partly through my friends. I was about 10 years of age at the time. Although I usually indulged in this vice in company, my heart glowed for a girl in school until I was 14, to such an extent that I felt hot and cold as soon as I saw her. After I started secondary school, I got to know my room-mates. We often slept in threes, even fours, in the same bed and satisfied each other's sexual desires with our hands. When we were about 16, we often got together with teacher candidates, and after some time, one of them, aged about 28, persuaded me to sleep with him. Of course, it didn't come to sleep, but the night was sacrificed to lust. The next day I was disgusted by the man and despite all his love concessions, I was unable to have relations with him a second time. I was ashamed of such an aged man. I only kept company with my room-mates, and mutual onanism was the order of the day. The leading figure among us was a young, strong lad from rich parents who often ordered us to forcefully perform onanism on one of us or to lie down in bed with him. Despite all his brutality, I was very fond of the young man, and he also felt a warm affection for me. Since I was destined to be a merchant from the beginning, I went to W. from secondary school to work in a large speciality shop. I was not yet 17 years of age at the time. Strangely enough, my urge for masturbation ceased completely. I went to the theatre now and then and made the acquaintance of a girl from the demimonde. I still had a liking for handsome men, but I did not feel the need to have sexual relations with them. The relationship with the aforementioned girl soon became more intimate. I thought myself to be a handsome, dashing fellow and felt flattered by the girl's obligingness. She lived in one of the first-class brothels, and in a short time I was a frequent and welcome guest in that house. I had sexual intercourse with the girl for almost 17 months, one or two nights a week. The girl was fond of me and never accepted anything from me by way of compensation. From W. I went to one of the first trading towns. I had the opportunity to get into society through my brother-in-law, and although I danced a lot, I mostly sought out gentlemen's company. After a stay of about six months, I came to know an older urning, and from that time on, the passion that had lain dormant for almost two years awoke in me. We only masturbated together, but the urge was kindled, and I enjoyed handsome men more than ever, especially muscular and beardless ones. This so-called friend introduced me to several of his acquaintances, praised me like a fine piece of merchandise, and soon I came to be the common property of many. My social intercourse often brought me together with military men, and I very soon fell in love with a young lieutenant. My love was not reciprocated, but only in friendship. I often pondered for a long time how I could trick my lover into sleeping with me.

After much manoeuvring, I succeeded in my plan. One evening when I was walking home, I told him that I had forgotten my gate key and that I couldn't ring the bell at such a late hour because of the noise of the dogs.

Friend H. invited me to sleep with him; I was trembling with excitement. After we undressed and I saw my dear strapping friend climb into bed, I was so ashamed of my intention that I absolutely refused to lie down with him and ended up sleeping alone on the couch. I was ashamed because I knew that my intention was wrong and that I would jeopardise the friendship. Later on, I did not have any more such feelings towards my friend, but he had all my love. During this time, I sometimes consorted with urnings, but always felt remorse after satisfying my lust. In order to throw sand in the eyes of my friends, I went to a brothel several times and also performed the sexual act with one of the women several times. I felt pleasure, but not as much as with a man. When I left this city, my love for my friend was the same, even though I had become quite immersed in the abominations of vice. It made me feel just as good to have a friend who was so morally high above me, despite my depravity.

Once back home, I naturally had to keep a low profile as much as possible in order to protect my family from disgrace and not ruin my existence. On the occasion of a conversation, I had the opportunity to invite one of my acquaintances, for whom it was too late and too far to go home, to stay with me, but I only enjoyed sleeping together, as I always had the consequences of carelessness in mind. I made do with masturbation. A new turning point in my life was brought about by a well-known singer who aroused my interest as an artist and as a person. I am a great lover of music and a special admirer of Richard Wagner. In Germany, I was often privileged to be able to admire the above artist; when I saw him there, my caution was over. I looked for an opportunity and found it. My newly acquired friend was more versed in the matter than I and fanned my affection to glowing flames of love. I followed him in everything and, at his request, abstained from all further contact for months. We saw each other almost every fortnight, made love and went on longer trips. Gradually, the thought often rose in me that my friend was taking love a little too casually, and my love became cooler. Our get-togethers became less frequent, and in the end all that remained was friendship, which we still maintain today. Now came another time of being alone, another time of masturbation. I went to Vienna more often now, about twice a year, made acquaintances, was also taken to the Central Bathhouse, which fully deserves the name male brothel. I know that I am not a hair's breadth better than the visitors to the aforementioned baths, but I had never encountered anything so disgusting in terms of lechery and such a gathering of like-minded people; I could not bring myself to stay in this bathing room any longer. Through the recommendation of my friend, I received many a visit in the last few years; I only accepted men with whom I could also show myself in the street, as I detest anything ordinary. I would like to mention one more case. During a visit to Vienna, I promenaded in the evening on a well-known path near the city park. I had never had to deal with a soldier before and decided to amuse myself with one for a fee. I soon met a handsome young soldier who had gone out to earn money. Of course, he suspected my intention and suggested that we go to an inn first. We had a drink together, and when I saw that he was only pursuing this service out of necessity, my desires immediately disappeared; I did my utmost to obliterate the impression that the way we became acquainted must have made on him, and we parted late that night without anything improper happening between us. In the course of the last two-and-a-half years, I became acquainted with a young lady, feeling not outright love, but only affection for her intellectual abilities. Since, in my position as a merchant with a large household, I am actually forced to acquire a wife, I decided to take the serious step that was so daring for me and became engaged to the lady mentioned. There came moments, even hours of regret, and yet I thought and hoped that a marriage could tear me out of my condition. At the beginning of my engagement, I indulged less in masturbation and even had, I think a few times when I held my bride, such excited feelings that my penis was in a stiff state.

The relationship came to an end due to various circumstances that do not belong here. My fiancée, who, by the way, was not at all beautiful, still loves me in the same way and, as I learned from her relatives, wants to wait until all obstacles have been overcome. When the relationship was dissolved, I felt pain in the first place; later I told myself it was better that way; I might have made the poor girl quite unhappy. My greatest joy would have been to have one or two children, and I have often regretted having wasted so much energy in vain instead of having fathered a child, even if it was out of wedlock.

The latter time passed in the usual way. I received many a gentleman sent to me, made the acquaintance of a like-minded young man with whom I had many sexual encounters and also gave myself up to passive pederasty: I am disgusted by active pederasty. About four weeks ago, I received another visit from a young man. We stayed in my flat and satisfied each other with our hands. I liked the young man from the first moment, and I did not seem unpleasant to him either. Since he was a guest at the spa and lived nearby, our visits to each other were repeated quite often. As time went by, my affection changed into such passionate love as I had never known. I complied with his wish to practise active pederasty with him, but I was unable to do so repeatedly. Even the last night we spent together, I could only perform the act with great difficulty. And yet my friend is the most precious thing I possess. I am impressed by his extraordinary education, his speech, his masculine behaviour, in short, everything. He is decidedly too good for me to perform a sexual act, although he is only for that matter. It would be my greatest wish if he and I could be put on the right track so that we could cultivate a true, noble friendship without any ulterior motives. I do not feel happy in spite of love, because I have to tell myself that my passion, my unhappy state, outrides this love. I would give a lot if my friend won me as a friend in the normal way.

These are the main features of my existence. In describing my childhood, I have overlooked the fact that as a little boy I liked to do my little sister's hair, wished I could dress myself in beautiful clothes in order to be seen, was not averse to playing with dolls, but did not enjoy female handicrafts. A younger brother of mine also seems to be addicted to masturbation.

No one in my family suspects my pathological condition, nor do any of my local friends. I am of medium height, strongly built, have a lot of hair all over my body, especially on my chest, have a moderately deep voice and am generally in a cheerful mood. My circle of friends consists of young people who are not like me. I have a somewhat soft disposition and can see neither man nor animal suffering. I like everything in nature, and I am also a keen tourist. I have had only one pollution in my life, and that was before I started taking daily baths.

I think my gait is a little strange, almost floating, but my gestures and manner of speaking do not suggest such a degeneration of sexual feeling. Strangely enough, I have a reputation here as a girl-hunter, which is perhaps due to the fact that two years ago I got a girl for myself under rather conspicuous circumstances. I also practised coitus and was satisfied that the girl spread the news quite a bit. How I would behave towards a female today I don't know, probably shameful for me. My genitals are normal, but I think that even though I rarely indulge in masturbation now, my sexual performance has gone downhill.

I don't dislike women's company at the moment, but I prefer to be in jolly gentlemen's company. I smoke heavily, drink a lot and hate with all my soul everything that is pretentious and unmanly about men. Little boys leave me cold, but young people of 18 interest me. I have not yet seduced anyone, because fear and shame have held me back.

This is my general confession. I never thought I would speak out to such an extent to a man who is not on our side. But I have written a lot from my heart with what I have said today. Reading your great work really made my heart feel good; contempt hurts so much, especially when one deserves only pity instead. It is through this base sexual instinct that we ourselves are most punished. I am not at all in favour of granting our passion so many rights by law, only I would like to see the public judgement softened for us unfortunates. A 'yuck', as I have often had to hear about others, always rings in my ears for a long time and always makes it clear to me how we are judged by society.

The drowning man is clutching at straw. Hopefully I will have a solid point of reference that will not let me sink in the pool of misery and contempt.

9.3 PS6 (1891) Bb 108, 239–40

R: *PS7 (1892) Bb 133, PS8 (1893) Bb 133, PS9 (1894) Bb 129*

My father was once struck by a stroke but is cured except for slight distortion of the face. My mother was very anaemic and melancholic. Both suffered badly from haemorrhoids, and my father attributed his back pains to them, from which he suffered from time to time, even after his marriage.

I am, if I may put it that way, a passive character. As a child, I indulged in all sorts of fantasies (some religious). I suffered from bed-wetting and was said to have played with my genitals in my sleep, which is why my father tied my hands to the bed! (I was still a child at that time and did not masturbate.) I was always very shy and awkward in relationships. I began masturbating when I was about 14 or 15. The urge and longing towards women associated with the awakening sexual feeling was actually only of a platonic nature; I also lacked contact with ladies. When I was about 18 years of age, I tried to satisfy my sexual needs in a natural way, more out of curiosity than out of an inner urge. Without ever having felt any inclination towards a woman, I satisfied my need through sexual intercourse as often as I could.

Soon after the onset of puberty, I had come to look very anaemic and much older than I was. Now, however, melancholy thoughts and strange ideas were added. It was a delight to me to imagine myself as degraded as possible. It may be of interest if I add that at that time I was struggling with religious doubts and only later found the courage to place myself above religion. I fell in love with young men. At first, I opposed these ideas, but later, they were so powerful that I came to be a true urning. Women seemed to me like people of the second class. I was in a dismal condition. Weariness of life and misanthropic impulses nestled in my sick soul. One day I read: '*Was will das werden*?'[2] And before I knew it, I was a social democrat, but an ideal one. Life had value for me again, for I had an ideal: the peaceful struggle for the social uplift of the proletarians. This brought about a powerful revolution in me. As in my best days (at the age of 16, 17), I became enthusiastic about art, especially drama. I immediately wrote a play and a farce and rolled great ideas around in my head. I read a remark by Schlegel about Sophocles, who owed his energy, creative power and music to his physical exercises and his artistic temperament. The passage 'The dramatist must first and foremost be intellectually intact' was very hard on my soul, for my contrary sexual feelings could not possibly come from a completely healthy mind.

I thought of having myself treated hypnotically, but shame prevented me from doing so. Now I told myself that I was a terrible weakling for having so little confidence in myself, and I took it upon myself earnestly to suppress my urning urges. At the same time, I fought my nervousness through a purposeful way of life. I rowed, crammed, spent a lot of time in the fresh air and had the joy of feeling like a completely different person when I woke up. When I think of the time from the age of 20 to 26, it was as if a completely strange and horrifying person had lived in my skin throughout that time.

I am astonished that the most handsome horseman, the tautest barman arouses almost no interest in me; even the muscular stonemasons leave me cold. It disgusts me to think that such people had ever seemed beautiful to me. My self-esteem increases; although I am very good-natured, and I am a thoroughly active character. My appearance has improved steadily since my twentieth year. I now look completely in keeping with my age. I do have relapses in my urges, but I suppress them vigorously. I satisfy my libido only through coitus and hope that with a further purposeful way of life, my desire will also increase.

9.4 NF (1891) Bb 2, 102–10

R: *PS7 (1892) Bb 110, PS8 (1893) Bb 110*

I am 31 years of age and an official in a factory in Poland. My parents are healthy and have nothing pathological about them. My paternal grandfather is said to have been brain-damaged; my maternal grandmother died melancholic, one of my mother's cousins was an alcoholic, several other blood relatives are not psychologically normal.

I was four years of age when my sex drive stirred. A man in his twenties who played with us children and took us in his arms aroused in me the desire to embrace him and kiss him fervently. This urge for a sensual kiss on the mouth is characteristic of me, since it is now the main stimulus for my sexual satisfaction. I felt a similar impulse in about my ninth year. A man, ugly and dirty, with a red beard also awakened in me this desire to kiss him. Here, for the first time, I experienced a characteristic that is still present in me today, namely, the peculiar sensual attraction of the common, even the dirty, in the clothing and behaviour of another person.

At grammar school, from the age of 11 to 15, I came to feel a passion for a comrade. It would have been my greatest desire to embrace him and kiss him mouth to mouth. I was sometimes seized by a desire for him that I do not feel more strongly towards people I now love. However, I don't think I had erections until around the age of 13.

During these years, as I said, I only had the desire to embrace and kiss; the desire to see or even touch the sexual parts of others was completely absent. I was a completely unspoilt, naive boy, didn't know the meaning of 'erection' until I was 15, and I didn't even dare kiss my lover because I felt I was doing something strange.

I did not feel the need to masturbate, and I was also lucky enough not to be tempted to do so by any older friends. In general, I have never masturbated until now. I feel a certain reluctance to do so.

Between the ages of 14 and 15, I became attracted to a number of boys, some of whom I still like today. I was very much in love with a boy whom I had never spoken to, but I was happy just to meet him on the street.

That my passions were of a thoroughly sensual nature is evident from the fact that even when I pressed and cajoled my beloved's hands, I got a violent erection. But it would always have been my greatest pleasure to embrace and kiss on the mouth; I did not desire anything else. I didn't know that what I felt was sexual love, only that I told myself it was impossible for me alone to feel such stimuli.

Until I was fifteen, I had never been aroused by a woman, but then one evening, while I was alone in the room with our maid, I felt the same desire as I felt towards many a boy; I first joked with her, and when I saw that she liked to kiss me, I covered her with kisses; I felt a lust that I rarely feel now. We kissed mouth to mouth, and after about 10 minutes I had pollution. I satisfied myself like this two or three times a week, and soon I began a similar relationship with one of our cooks and other maids. Ejaculation occurred after about 10 minutes of prolonged kissing.

In the meantime, I had been taking dancing lessons, and for the first time I was attracted to a fine girl. This love disappeared quite soon, however, and I then fell in love with another girl whom I never met, but at the sight of whom I felt a similar attraction to the young boys, not just the purely sensual, brutal glow as I usually felt towards girls. At this time, my urge for girls had reached its peak; I was attracted to about the same percentage of girls as I was to young men. I satisfied my sensuality, as mentioned above, by kissing the maid, with subsequent pollution; this is how I spent the time between the ages of 16 and 18. The departure of our maids deprived me of the opportunity for sensual gratification.

There came a time of two to three years during which I had to renounce sexual pleasure; I liked girls less and less, and now that I had grown up, I was ashamed to spend time with maids. It was not possible for me to acquire a mistress, for despite my age, I was strictly supervised by my parents and only met a few young men, so little was my independence. As the urge for women diminished, the attraction for young boys increased.

Since I had had many nocturnal pollutions since the age of 16, with dreams partly of women and partly of men, which weakened me greatly and depressed me completely, I wanted to put an end to them through normal coitus.

Scruples, however, and the belief that prostitutes did not attract me, kept me away from the brothel until I was 21. For two to three years, I fought a daily battle (but if there had been male brothels, no scruples would have prevented me from going). Finally, I went to the brothel; I did not even manage to get an erection, on the one hand because the girl, although she was unusually fresh and pretty for a brothel madam, did not excite me, but especially because she did not want to kiss me on the mouth. I was extremely depressed and thought I was impotent; three weeks later I visited another prostitute, who immediately brought me to erection with her kiss; she was of buxom form, wide lips, much more sensual than the first. After only three minutes, just kissing mouth to mouth led to ejaculation

([*LATIN: outside the entrance*], of course). So it was only after I had been with prostitutes about seven times that I made attempts at coitus.

The first time I didn't get an erection at all, because the girl was cold, and the second time I ejaculated too early. In general, the first few times I felt a little disgust [*LATIN: introducing my penis*], and even after I had succeeded in having normal coitus, I felt no stimulus from it. The satisfaction of lust happens through kisses on the mouth, this alone is the most important thing for me; coitus only serves as something secondary to the more intimate embrace. Mere coitus, no matter how much the woman stimulates me, would be indifferent to me without kissing; indeed, my erection usually subsides or does not arise if the woman does not want to kiss on the mouth. I cannot kiss every woman, but only those whose face attracts me; a strumpet who is repugnant to me even at the sight of her does not bring me into ardour by all the kissing, which then only disgusts me.

I have been visiting brothels for four years, about every 10–14 days; only rarely do I still fail at coitus, since I have got to know myself and know immediately when I choose the prostitute whether she will excite me or leave me cold. However, just lately it has happened again that I thought the woman would excite me, yet every erection was missing. This was especially true when I had had to forcefully suppress my urge for men the days before.

In the early days, when I went to the brothel, the sensation of lust was very slight; only very few times did I have true desire (as I used to when kissing). Now, on the other hand, I usually feel a strong sensation of lust. Ordinary brothels have a special attraction for me, because lately the vulgarity of the women, the dark entrance, the pale glow of the lanterns, the whole environment exerts a special attraction on me, especially because my sensuality is unconsciously incited by the frequent intercourse of soldiers in such places and, as it were, gives the woman a certain attraction. If I then find a woman whose face excites me, I can feel very strong desire.

Apart from prostitutes, my desires can be aroused by peasant girls, maids, workers, common girls, and in general those in common clothing. Red cheeks, thick lips, buxom body shapes are especially pleasing to me. I am indifferent to fine ladies and young ladies.

My pollutions are mostly without voluptuous sensations, often during dreams of men, extremely rarely, almost never, of women. As can be seen from the latter, despite regular coitus, I still have a drive for young men. Yes, I can say that it has only increased, and to a significant degree. If girls are completely unattractive to me immediately after coitus, the kiss of a likeable woman could immediately bring back my erection; it is precisely during the first days after coitus that young men seem most desirable to me.

In general, sexual intercourse with women does not satisfy all my sensual needs. I have days when I frequently find myself with an erection with a powerful urge for young men, then come calmer days with moments of complete indifference to every woman and latent urges for men.

Otherwise, too much sensual calm makes me sad again, especially when such calm follows moments of suppressed excitement, and only when the thought of beloved young men causes me erections do I feel in an elevated mood again. The calm then changes again into great nervousness; I feel depressed, sometimes have a headache (especially after a repressed erection), and this nervousness very often increases to an uncontrollable restlessness which I then try to calm by coitus.

A significant change in my sexual life took place last year when I was able to experience male love for the first time. Despite pleasurable female coitus (i.e. more correctly, pleasurable kissing with ejaculation), my urge for young men did not give me any peace. I decided to go to a brothel frequented by many soldiers and, if the worst came to the worst, to buy myself a soldier. I was lucky enough to immediately meet a like-minded man who, despite his much lower rank, was not unworthy of me in character and behaviour. What I felt (or still feel) with this young man is different from what I feel with women. The sensual pleasure is no greater than with prostitutes, whose kiss and embrace excite me extraordinarily; on the other hand, I can feel lust with him at any time, and there is a feeling towards him that is lacking with women. Unfortunately, I have only been able to hug and kiss him about eight times.

Although we have been separated for many months, as he has been transferred to a garrison in Hungary, we have not forgotten each other and correspond regularly. In order to possess him, I dared to go to a brothel and embrace him there at the risk of being betrayed.

At the beginning of our acquaintance there came a time when I heard nothing more from him, since he, for his part, did not consider me reliable. During these weeks, I endured an agony and torment that brought me to a dejection and anxious restlessness such as I had never felt before. To have hardly found a lover, only to have to renounce him again, seemed to me the supreme torment. When, thanks to my efforts, we came together again, my joy was boundless; indeed, I was so excited that when I saw him again, I did not reach ejaculation during his embrace despite my sensual lust.

Sexual intercourse with him consisted of kisses and embraces, and he was also allowed to play with my penis (whereas the touching of it by the hand of a woman is unbearable to me, and I never allow a woman such a touch). It should be noted, by the way, that when I am with my lover, I immediately get an erection; a handshake is enough, even the sight of him. I walked with him for hours during the evening, not for a moment tired of his company despite his social position, which was inferior to mine; I felt happy with him, and sexual satisfaction was only the crowning glory of our love. Although I had finally found the like-minded man I had been seeking for so long and was finally allowed to measure manly love, I did not become insensitive to women, and I visited brothels when the urge plagued me too violently. I had hoped to spend this winter in the city of my beloved, but unfortunately this was impossible, and I am now forced to be separated from him for the foreseeable future. However, we will try to see each other, even if only temporarily, and even if only once or twice a year; in any case, I hope that in the future we will perhaps be together again for a longer time. So for this winter I am once again forced to remain without a like-minded friend. I had resolved not to go in search of other urnings again because of the danger of being discovered, but this is impossible for me, for sexual intercourse with women does not satisfy me; on the other hand, my desire for young men is growing more and more. I am sometimes afraid of myself, that by asking all the prostitutes whether they know of any like-minded person, I might one day be discovered. Nevertheless, I cannot refrain from seeking a youth of my sensibility; indeed, I know I will buy a soldier for myself, if necessary, although I am clearly aware of the daring of such an undertaking.

I can no longer remain without male love; without such love I will forever remain in disharmony with myself. My ideal would be to associate with a number of like-minded people, although I would even be satisfied to associate freely with one lover. I could easily do without women if I had regular male satisfaction, but I believe that at times I would also embrace a woman in longer intervals for a change, for my nature is a complete hermaphrodite in psycho-sexual terms (in sexual matters I desire women and love and desire young men). If there were marriage between men, I believe I would not shy away from a lifelong union, though such a consecration seems to me something impossible. On the one hand, even if a woman were very attractive to me, I would very soon lose this attraction for regular intercourse, and then any sexual pleasure would be, if not impossible, then certainly without pleasure for me; on the other hand, however, true love would be lacking towards the woman, this attraction, as I feel it towards beloved young men, and which even makes mere non-sensual intercourse seem desirable to me.

A constant companionship with a young man who would otherwise please me physically, but who would also agree with me intellectually, who would understand all my feelings and at the same time share my intellectual views and aspirations, would seem to me to be the greatest happiness.

The young men who appeal to me must be between 18 and 28 years of age; with increasing age, the age limit of the young men who appeal to me has also increased. Otherwise, I can be attracted to a wide variety of builds. The main role, even if not almost exclusively, is played by the face, more blondes than brunettes excite me, they must not be bearded, they must only have a small, not thick moustache, or none at all. For the rest, I can only say that I like certain categories of faces. Faces with large straight noses and pale cheeks are excluded, although there are exceptions. I look with pleasure at regiments of soldiers, and I like many a man in a soldier's uniform who would leave me cold in civilian clothing.

Just as I am often attracted to a certain vulgar dress (especially light-coloured jackets) among women, I am also attracted to military costume. Going to dance halls, ordinary taverns where many soldiers are to be found, mingling with the crowd of soldiers and trying to win the boys I like for a kiss and an embrace, even if in an intellectual and social respect, every vulgarity in speech and behaviour is repugnant to me; this mingling with soldiers would, of course, only be an excitement for the senses. With young men of a better class, sensual desire comes to the fore less violently.

What I have said about the attraction of certain clothing is not to be understood in the sense that they excite me in and of themselves. This attraction only means that the clothing can contribute to intensifying or emphasising the attraction caused by the face, whereas otherwise perhaps the very same face would not have attracted me to the same extent. I can say the same, only in a slightly different sense, of the smell of cigar smoke. With indifferent persons, the smell of cigars is more repugnant to me than pleasant, but with persons I like sexually, it is arousing. The kiss of a harlot smelling of cigar smoke increases the attraction (especially because it comes to me, even if partly unconsciously, as a reminder of a man's kiss). I also liked to kiss my lover when he had just smoked. (It should be noted that I have never smoked a cigar or cigarette myself, nor have I ever even tried it.)

I am tall and slender, my face is masculine, my eyes are restless and my whole figure often has something girlish about it. My health leaves much to be desired; it is probably very much influenced by my sexual anomaly; as already mentioned earlier, I am very nervous, and at times I also have attacks of so-called brooding. I also have moments of terrible depression and melancholy, especially when I consider the difficulty of male satisfaction corresponding to my nature, as when I have been very sexually aroused and overcome the impulse when male satisfaction is impossible. In such states, depression is often paired with the entire absence of desire. I am diligent in my work, but often only fleetingly, as I am very inclined to work quickly, even fiercely. I am very interested in art and literature. Among poets and novelists, I am most attracted to those who describe refined feelings, peculiar passions, selected impressions; an artificial (or overly-artistic) style appeals to me. Likewise in music, the nervous, provocative music of Chopin, Schumann, Schubert, Wagner and so on is most appealing to me. Everything in art that is not only original but bizarre attracts me.

I do not love physical exercise and do not cultivate it.

My character is good-natured and compassionate. Despite the fact that I have to suffer so much with my anomaly, I do not feel unhappy that I love young men, but [I am unhappy] only insofar as the satisfaction of such love is considered unlawful and especially that I cannot obtain satisfaction without hindrance. I, myself, do not feel that the love of men is a vice, but I can understand why it is considered a vice. But since this love is considered criminal, I shall come to harmony with myself through the satisfaction of it, but never with the world of our time, and necessarily for that reason, I shall always be somewhat distempered; all the more so because I am an open character that hates every lie. This torment of always having to conceal everything within me has led me to confess my anomaly to a few friends, of whose taciturnity and at the same time of whose understanding I am certain. Although my situation sometimes seems sad to me because of the difficulty of satisfaction and the general disregard for male love, I am often downright vain to have such anomalous feelings. Of course, I will never marry; this seems to me no misfortune at all, although I love family life and until now have only spent my time with my family. I live in the hope that later I will have a lover permanently; I must get one, otherwise the future seems grey and dull to me, and all the goals one usually chases—honour, high position and so on—appear vain and unattractive.

Should this hope not be fulfilled, I know that I would not be able to devote myself to my profession with joy later on, and that I would be able to put everything aside in order to gain male love. I no longer have moral scruples about my abnormal inclination and have never worried about feeling attracted to young men. In general, I judge moral and immoral things according to my feelings, rather than according to fixed principles, because I am still caught up in scepticism and have not yet worked my way through to a fixed world view. So far, it seems to me that only what harms others, what I do not want to have done to myself, is bad and immoral, and in this direction, I can say that I try to interfere as little as possible with the rights of others, and I am able to feel lively indignation about an injustice done to others. How, on the other hand, love for men should be something immoral, I do not know; purposeless activity of the sexual instinct (if the immoral is to be seen in the purposeless, the unnatural) is also present in intercourse with prostitutes, and even in marriage in the use of means of protection against procreation, and it seems to me that sexual intercourse with men must come to be placed on the same level with all sexual intercourse which does not aim at procreation. But whether only sexual satisfaction that pursues this purpose should be moral seems questionable to me. It is true that sexual gratification not directed to procreation is contrary to nature, but whether such gratification does not serve other purposes unknown to us is uncertain, and even if it were purposeless, its reprehensibility does not follow (since it is not at all certain that the standard of a moral act is its expediency).

That the present prejudice will disappear I am sure, and I am certain that one day such individuals who feel manly love will come to be accorded the right of unhindered love. Incidentally, for the possibility of such recognition, think only of the Greeks and the friendships of that time, which were nothing other than sexual love; think of the fact that in spite of such unnatural fornication, which is practised by the greatest minds, the Greeks are still mentioned today as unrivalled models in intellectual and aesthetic terms and are recommended for imitation.

I have even thought of having my anomaly cured by hypnotism. If I submitted to hypnotism, which I doubt could do anything, I would have to be sure that I would really come to love women permanently. For even if I cannot satisfy myself with men, I would rather feel this capacity for exuberant desire and love, even if unsatisfied, than be completely insensitive. So I am left with the hope that I will also come to find the opportunity to satisfy the love I desire and which makes me happy, while I will not prefer a mere withdrawal of homosexual feelings without a simultaneous substitution of equivalent heterosexual ones to the present state.

Finally, I would like to comment on various statements by urnings in the published biographies that I, at least, find it very difficult to recognise as like-minded. Although I have described my sexual anomalies in some detail, the following remarks seem important to me for a better understanding of my condition.

Lately I have renounced [*LATIN: penetration with penis*] and contented myself with coitus [*LATIN: between the thighs of a girl*]. Ejaculation occurred more quickly than with [*LATIN: genital conjunction*], and I also felt a certain sensation of lust on the penis itself. If this kind of sexual intercourse was quite agreeable to me, this is perhaps partly due to the fact that in this kind of sexual pleasure the difference of sex is quite indifferent, and I probably came to unconsciously remember male embrace. But this recollection would have been quite unconscious, though darkly felt, in that I had not, thanks to my imagination, enjoyed it, but directly through kissing the woman's mouth.

I feel that the attraction that brothels and prostitutes exert on me is beginning to fade, but I know that certain women will always be able to excite me through their kiss. Yet no woman is desirable to me to the extent that I would be able to overcome any difficulties to obtain a wife, and there never will be one while even the danger of possible discovery and disgrace can only with difficulty keep me from seeking the embrace of a man. So I let myself be tempted to buy a soldier from a prostitute in the latter times. The lust was very great, but the feeling of satisfaction afterwards was especially uplifting for me. For the next few days, I felt strengthened (with erections possible at any time) and, although I can no longer meet the soldier, I am reassured by the thought that I will dare to buy another one, but I would only be completely satisfied if I found a like-minded person of my standing and education.

I have not yet mentioned that, while a female body (except for the face) and female sexual parts leave me completely cold (touching the latter with my hand would be disgusting to me), touching the male member while kissing mouth to mouth is desirable to me, and even kissing a very likeable man would have no disgust for me.

Masturbation, as already mentioned, would be quite impossible for me.

9.5 PS7 (1892) Bb 94, 194–7

R: *PS8 (1893) Bb 94, PS10 (1898) Bb 104*

I am a civil servant and come from a family that, as far as I know, is unencumbered; my father died of an acute illness, and my mother, who is alive, is rather 'nervous'. One sister has become very intensely religious for some years.

I, myself, am tall and make a thoroughly masculine impression in speech, gait and bearing. The only illnesses I have had are measles, but from the age of 13 I have suffered from so-called nervous headaches.

My sexual life began in my thirteenth year, when I met a slightly older boy, with whom we amused ourselves by touching each other's genital organs. In my fourteenth year, I had my first ejaculation. Seduced into masturbation by two older schoolmates, I indulged in it partly with others, partly alone, but in the latter case always with the thought of persons of the female sex in mind. My [*LATIN: sexual desire*] was very great, as it still is today. Later, I tried to attach myself to a pretty, vigorous maid with very firm [*LATIN: breasts. I got only so far that in my presence she would bare the upper part of her body and allow me to kiss her mouth and breasts, while she herself took my very erect penis by her hand and rubbed it.*] No matter how vehemently I demanded coitus, she would not permit it, but finally only allowed me to touch her sexual parts.

When I got to university, I went to a brothel and I was able to function without any effort.

But then an event occurred that brought about a change in me. One evening, I accompanied a friend home and, a little tipsy as I was, grabbed him [*LATIN: by the genitals*]. He resisted only a little; I then went to his room with him; we masturbated and from then on did this mutual masturbation quite frequently; it even came to [*LATIN: penetration of the penis into the mouth*] with subsequent ejaculation. The only strange thing was that I was not in the least in love with this person, but passionately in love with another of my friends, in whose vicinity I never felt the slightest sexual excitement, whom I never associated with sexual processes in my thoughts. My visits to brothels, where I was a welcome guest, became less frequent; I found a substitute in my friend and did not long for sexual intercourse with women.

We never practised sodomy; the word never came to mind between us. Since the beginning of this relationship with my friend, I masturbated more; naturally, thoughts of females receded more and more into the background. I thought of young, handsome, lusty men with as large penises as I could. Boys aged 16 to 25 without beards were my favourite, but they had to be handsome and clean. I was particularly attracted to young workers with trousers made of so-called Manchester fabric or English leather, especially bricklayers.

People of the same class hardly excite me at all, but I feel a clear sexual arousal at the sight of such a strapping young man from the people. Touching such trousers, opening them, grasping the penis and kissing the boy seem to me to be of the highest attraction. My receptivity to female stimuli is somewhat dulled, but I am always potent in sexual intercourse with a woman, especially if she has well-developed [*LATIN: breasts*], without using fantasy images. I have never attempted to abuse a young worker or the like for my unpleasant desires, nor will I do so, but I very often feel the desire to do so. Sometimes I hold on to the image of such a fellow and then masturbate at home.

I have no sense of female occupation at all. I am moderately fond of women's company. I dislike dancing. I take a lively interest in the fine arts. The fact that I sometimes have contra-sexual feelings is, I believe, partly a consequence of great comfort, which prevents me from having any kind of relationship with a girl, as it is too much trouble for me: always visiting brothels is repugnant to me for aesthetic reasons; so I fall into the tiresome masturbation, from which it is very difficult for me to refrain.

I have told myself a hundred times that, in order to be able to have completely normal sexual feelings, I must, above all, suppress the almost indomitable passion for the unfortunate masturbation, this aberration which is so repugnant to my aesthetic feelings; I have resolved so often to fight against this passion with all the strength of my will; I have not yet succeeded. Instead of seeking satisfaction in a natural way when the sexual urge stirred in me particularly violently, I preferred to masturbate because I felt that I would get more pleasure from it.

Experience has taught me that I am always potent with girls, without any effort and without the aid of images of male genitals, with the exception of a single case in which I did not achieve ejaculation because the female in question—it was in a brothel—was not stimulating. I cannot refrain from the thought and the heavy self-reproach that the contrasexuality is a consequence of excessive masturbation, and this has such a depressing effect on me because I have to tell myself that I hardly feel the strength within me to completely renounce this vice by my own free will.

As a result of the sexual relationship with a fellow student and long-time school friend mentioned in my letter—which only came about during our time at university, after we had been on friendly terms for seven years—the urge for unnatural satisfaction of the libido has come to me considerably stronger.

Please allow me to tell you about an episode that gave me a lot of trouble for months. In the summer of 1882, I met a fellow student who was six years younger than I and who had been recommended to me and my acquaintances along with several others. Very soon I felt a deep interest in the handsome, immensely proportioned, slim and healthy-looking man, which, after several weeks of social intercourse, developed into an intense feeling of friendship, then into passionate love and a tormenting sense of jealousy. I soon realised that I was strongly influenced by sensual impulses, and no matter how firmly I resolved to keep myself in check towards this person—who, apart from anything else, I held in such high esteem because of his excellent character—one night, when we were sitting in my flat with a bottle of champagne after having drunk a lot of beer and were drinking to good, true and lasting friendship, I succumbed to an irresistible desire to press him against me and so on.

When I saw him again the next day, I was so ashamed that I could not look him in the eye. I felt the bitterest remorse for my offence and reproached myself most vehemently for having so defiled this friendship, which was supposed to be and remain pure and noble. In order to prove to him that I had only been momentarily carried away, I urged him to go on a journey with me at the end of the semester; after some reluctance, the reasons for which were only too clear to me, he agreed; we slept in the same room for several nights without me making the slightest attempt to repeat that action. I wanted to talk to him about what had happened that night, but I couldn't manage it; when we were separated the following semester, I couldn't bring myself to write to him about the matter in question, and when I visited him in X in March, I felt the same way again. And yet I felt the most urgent need to clarify this dark point through an open discussion. In October of this year, I was again in X, and this time I found the courage for an unreserved discussion. I asked him for forgiveness, which he gladly granted me; indeed, I even asked him why he did not offer me resolute resistance at that time, to which he replied that he had partly left me to my own devices out of courtesy, and partly because he had been quite drunk and was thus caught up in a certain apathy. I explained my condition to him in detail, also gave him *Psychopathia Sexualis* to read and expressed to him the firm hope that I would succeed by my own strength in completely and permanently mastering my unnatural urges. Since this discussion, the relationship between that friend and myself has been the most pleasant and gratifying imaginable; the friendly feelings on both sides are intimate, true and, I hope, lasting.

If I should not see an improvement in my abnormal condition, I would probably decide to submit myself completely to your treatment, all the more so since, after a careful study of your work, I cannot count myself in the category of the so-called urnings. Rather, I have the firm conviction, or at least the hope, that the firmest will, supported and guided by expert treatment, can turn me into a normal human being.

Notes

1. Neurasthenia or cerebral asthenia was a poorly defined psychiatric diagnosis of this period in history. It was characterised by tiredness, lack of energy, headache and irritableness.
2. This was the novel *Was will das werden?: Roman in neun Büchern* by Friedrich Spielhagen. Spielhagen was one of the leading authors of his age and his works advanced a radical democratising philosophy.

CHAPTER 10

In Search of a Cure

10.1 PS7 (1892) Bb 109, 241–5

R: *PS8 (1893) Bb 109*

I was born in the year 1868. Both my parents' families are healthy. At any rate, mental illness has never occurred in them. My father was a merchant; he is now 65 years of age and has been nervous for years, especially inclined to melancholy. Before his marriage, my father is said to have been an enthusiastic pleasure seeker. My mother is healthy, although not very strong. I have two healthy siblings.

I, myself, was sexually developed at a very early age and, around the age of 14, had to deal with wet dreams to such an extent that I became frightened. I can no longer say under what circumstances these occurred, and in particular what kinds of dreams were associated with them. The fact is that for years, I have felt sexually attracted only to men, and despite all my energy and terrible struggle, I cannot conquer this unnatural urge which is so repugnant to me. In the first years of my life, I am said to have suffered many serious illnesses, so much so that people repeatedly feared for my life. That is probably why I was spoiled and very pampered. I was always in my room a lot, preferred playing with dolls to playing with soldiers and generally preferred quiet games in my room to noisy street games. At the age of 10 I went to grammar school. Although I was very

D. Pretsell, *Queer Voices in the Works of Richard von Krafft-Ebing, 1883–1901*, Genders and Sexualities in History,
https://doi.org/10.1007/978-3-031-17331-8_10

lazy, I was one of the best pupils, because I learned very easily and was the favourite of my teachers. From my earliest childhood (age seven), I took pleasure in little girls. I remember that I had serious love affairs with them until I was 13 years of age, that I was jealous of those who socialised with them, that I enjoyed looking up the skirts of my sister's friends and the servants, that I got an erection when I touched the bodies of the girls I played with. But I can certainly remember that boys attracted and sexually aroused me just as early and powerfully. I always enjoyed reading and the theatre; I had a puppet theatre that I loved to play with, knew whole plays by heart, copied the actors I saw, especially choosing the female roles, and enjoyed dressing up in women's clothing.

As my sexual life awakened more strongly, my inclinations for boys gained the upper hand. I fell completely in love with my friends, had a lustful feeling when one of them I liked touched my body. I became very shy, refusing to go to gym class and swimming. I thought I was different from my friends and was embarrassed to undress in front of them. I took pleasure in looking at my friends' penises and got erections very easily. I only masturbated once in my youth. When a friend told me that one could have pleasure without women, I also tried it, but did not enjoy it. I also came across a book that warned me of the consequences of masturbation. I did not do it again after that one time. In my fourteenth or fifteenth year, I met two slightly younger boys who excited me sexually to the highest degree. I was completely in love with one of them in particular. I became sexually excited around him, restless when he wasn't with me, jealous of anyone who socialised with him, and self-conscious in his presence. He had no idea of my condition. I felt very unhappy, cried often and gladly, because then I felt relieved. But I could not understand this feeling of mine; I always felt that it was irregular. In particular, I was also unhappy that my ability to work suddenly diminished. I, who used to learn with ease, suddenly had the greatest difficulty; my thoughts were never focused. Only with the expenditure of all my energy did I manage to get anything into my head. I always had to learn aloud to keep my attention. My memory, previously excellent, often let me down. In spite of that I still remained a good pupil and am still considered a gifted person today, but I have terrible trouble memorising things. At that time, I put all my energy into freeing myself from this miserable state. I went swimming every day, did gymnastics, rode a lot and diligently visited the fencing ground, and also took great pleasure in all these activities. Even today I feel very comfortable on a horse, although I know nothing about horses and have no particular talent for physical exercise. I took great pleasure in socialising with my friends; I never missed a pub party, I smoked and was very popular. I spent a lot of time in pubs with female waitresses and enjoyed having fun with the waitresses, but without becoming sexually excited. My friends and teachers regarded me as a person who did a lot with women and was spoilt. Unfortunately, wrongly.

I went to university at the age of 19. I spent my first semester at B. University. I still have terrible memories of it today. My sexual need arose powerfully, and I walked around for hours at night, especially when I was turned on, looking for men. Fortunately, I found no one. The next morning, I was beside myself. In the second semester I went to M. This was my happiest time. I had nice friends, miraculously took a liking to women and was quite happy about it. I made love to a young, depraved girl with whom I spent wild nights, and I was extraordinarily powerful. I, who had previously been chaste, also had other relations with women. I felt fresh and good as never before after coitus. With women, I was not attracted by the figure, which I found unattractive—I don't know why—but I became acquainted with women whose touch immediately resulted in erection. This joy and happy state did not last long. I did the foolish thing of moving into a flat with a male friend. We had one bedroom. He was a very gifted, amiable and dangerous man to women, and it was these qualities that first attracted me to him. I only love very educated men, whereas uneducated, strong people can only excite me instantly, but not captivate me. Soon I fell in love with my friend. Now came the terrible time that destroyed my health. I slept in the same room as my friend, had to watch him undress before my eyes every day, and had to summon up all my energy not to betray myself. I became nervous, cried easily, and was jealous of anyone who had relations with my friend. I was still consorting with women, but could only bring myself to coitus with difficulty, which was disgusting to me, just like the woman herself. The same women who had previously excited me most vividly now left me cold. I followed my friend to W., where he met an acquaintance from earlier times, with whom he moved in together. I became jealous, sick with longing and love. At the same time, I again had relations with women, but only rarely and with difficulty did I manage to have sex. I became terribly disgruntled, close to madness. There was no more talk of working. I led a foolish, exhausting life and needed endless amounts of money, which I virtually threw out the window. Then I collapsed after six weeks and had to go to a hydropathic clinic, where I spent many months. I regained my senses there and soon became very popular, as I can be very funny and find a lot of pleasure socialising with educated ladies. I prefer married women to younger ones in conversation, but I am also very funny in gentlemen's company, at the beer table, in the bowling alley.

In this institution, I met a man of 29 who was obviously of a similar disposition as I. He wanted to embrace and kiss me, but I found him terribly disgusting, even though he excited me and his touch gave me erections that even led to ejaculation. One evening, he seduced me into mutual masturbation. I spent the most terrible night without sleep, was terribly disgusted by the experience, and I resolved never again to do such things with a man. For days I could not get any rest. It was appalling to me that the man had sexually aroused me despite all this and against my will; on the other hand, it gave me satisfaction that the same man was in love with me and obviously had to endure similar struggles as I had earlier. I learned how to keep him away from then on.

I went to various universities again, visited some hydropathic institutions with some success, but never lasting. I still fell in love with many a friend, but never as strongly as with the man in M. I no longer had sexual intercourse, neither with women—because I was incapable of it—nor with men, because I lacked the opportunity and forced myself to turn away from them. I still met my friend from M. often, we are now better friends than ever and he no longer upsets me, which I am extremely happy about. It's usually like this: if I haven't seen a person who excites me sexually for a long time, the sexual influence disappears.

I passed my exams with distinction. In the last year before the exam, I started to do it [masturbate]—that is, at the age of 23—because I didn't know any other way to satisfy my sex drive, which bothered me so much. However, I did it very seldom, as I was always disgusted and had sleepless nights afterwards. Only when I have drunk a lot do I lose all energy. I then walk around for hours, looking for men, which finally ends in masturbation, only to wake up the next day with a dull head and a terrible disgust for myself, and I walk around melancholically for days. As long as I am in control of myself, I try to fight against my nature with all my energy. It's terrible when you can't be calm with any friend, when every strapping soldier or butcher's boy makes you tremble and shake. It is terrible when night comes, and I lurk at the window to see if someone is urinating on the wall opposite and giving me the opportunity to look at his genitals. These dreams are horrible, and in addition, I am aware of the immorality, the punishability of my attitude and my desires. I have an aversion to myself that cannot be described. I consider my condition to be pathological. I cannot consider it to be innate, but I believe that the urge is instilled in me through a mistaken upbringing. My suffering makes me reckless and selfish; it robs me of any good-naturedness and any consideration for my family. I am moody and often driven to madness, often disgruntled, so that I hardly know how to help myself, and then very easily inclined to tears. And yet I have a disgust for sexual intercourse with men. One evening, when I came from the pub drunk and excited and was wandering around the promenade in this semi-conscious state and full of lust, I met a young man who seduced me into mutual masturbation. Although he excited me, I was beside myself after what had happened. Even today, when I pass by the place, I can't help feeling disgusted, and the other day, when I was riding by, I fell off the honest beast I knew so well, so disgusted was I by the memory of this unworthiness.

I love family and children, social intercourse and, according to my position in society, I am suited to maintain a household. I have to do without all this, and yet I cannot give up the hope of a cure. So I hover between hopeful cheerfulness and appalling hopelessness, neglecting job and family. I don't even want to get as far as getting married and starting a family. I only want to learn how to overcome the terrible inclination towards the male sex, to communicate calmly with my friends again and to learn to respect myself again.

No one has any idea of my condition. I am rather considered a terrible ladies' man, which reputation I try to maintain. I often try to establish a relationship with girls, for which I am frequently offered the opportunity. I have met many a girl who loved me and would have sacrificed her honour for me, but I cannot offer her any love and cannot grant her anything sexually. But I can love a man. I am only excited by men who are very young—that is, between 17 and 25 years of age, who do not have a full beard or preferably no beard at all. I can only love those who are very educated, decent and kind. I, myself, am short, very vain and frivolous, also very exalted, easily led by the people I like and whom I try to imitate in everything, but also very sensitive and easily offended by them. I attach great importance to appearances, love beautiful furnishings and clothing and can be impressed by a distinguished manner and elegant appearance. I am unhappy that my neurasthenic condition prevents me from doing and learning everything I would like to.

[KRAFFT-EBING: I met the patient in the autumn. He is without signs of degeneration, of thoroughly masculine physical build, though delicately

built and slight. Genitals quite normal. His outer appearance is distinguished and inconspicuous. He deeply laments his sexual perversion, from which he would like to rid himself of at all costs. In spite of the greatest efforts on the part of the doctor and the patient, only a very slight degree of hypnosis, insufficient for suggestive treatment, could be achieved.]

10.2 PS7 (1892) Bb 135, 326–9

R: *PS8 (1893) Bb 135, PS9 (1894) Bb 131*

[KRAFFT-EBING: Acquired contra-sexual feeling. Considerable improvement through hypnotic treatment. Mr. P., born 1863, factory official, comes from a distinguished patrician family in Central Germany, in which nervousness and insanity were frequent occurrences. His paternal great-grandfather and his sister died of insanity, his grandmother of apoplexy, his father's brother of insanity, his daughter of cerebral tuberculosis. Maternal mother was melancholic for years, maternal father mentally ill: mother's brother took his own life in a fit of mental disorder. The patient's father is very nervous. One older brother is severely neurasthenic with anomalies of the vita sexualis, *another is the subject of Observation 108 of the sixth edition of* Psychopathia Sexualis, *a third exhibits eccentric behaviour and is said to have fixed ideas, one sister is convulsive, another died of convulsions as a small child.*

The patient is afflicted, for already at an early age he was highly peculiar, irritable, irascible and gave the impression of being an abnormal person to those around him. Very early on, his vita sexualis *was revealed powerfully, and he satisfied it, without any seduction, through masturbation. From the age of 16, the young boy visited the brothels of the capital, using his free time on Sundays and holidays for this purpose. He copulated with pleasure, satisfying himself with masturbation during the weekdays. From the age of 20 and having become independent, the patient excessively used prostitutes, fell ill with* neurasthenia sexualis *and became relatively impotent and unsatisfied by coitus due to erectile dysfunction and [*LATIN: premature ejaculation*]. His* libido sexualis *became more powerful than ever and satisfied by masturbation. The patient met a young man at the beginning of 1888.]*

By his pleasing face, his ingratiating manner, by his beautiful external physical build, he acquired my very special affection. I wanted to talk to him and always looked forward to the moment when I saw him. I fell completely in love with him. With that, my love for women was extinguished. That man could excite me to such an extent that I felt my memory fade away in seconds, and I stuttered.

Soon afterwards I met a gentleman who was also very attractive and had decisive influence on my future life. He was man-loving. I confessed to him that I truly only felt disgust for the female sex and was attracted to men.

When I once asked my friend how he managed to get soldiers to surrender to him, he replied that the main thing was grit; anyone could be brought around. At the end of 1888, bearing these words in mind, I approached a fellow, an officer; I was greatly stimulated by him, although ejaculation never occurred. Since I saw that the soldier did not want to surrender easily, I gave up on him. [*LATIN: Another soldier who had once been admitted into my bedroom I asked to undress and lie down on my bed with me. After he had been asked, he did what I wanted and we each rubbed the other's penis.*]

Although I abused many people like this after this happy success, I was only in love, so to speak, with one. He was a very handsome lad of 17. His voice sounded so ingratiating to me, and his behaviour was so decently tender that I still can't forget him. In my dreams I was only preoccupied with beautiful young men and often couldn't sleep for long nights because of sensuality.

[KRAFFT-EBING: At the beginning of 1889, the patient's behaviour aroused suspicion of male love. A report threatening him frightened and upset him deeply, so much so that he planned suicide On the advice of the family doctor, he came to the capital. As the patient was incapable of renouncing his habitual cravings of his own accord, a hypnotic treatment was initiated. It only achieved a slight numbness and was not very successful compared to the seduction of former lovers in whose vicinity the patient was.

At that time, the patient still lacked moral seriousness. The situation improved in the face of the ideas of dismayed relatives and the spectre of a real threat of judicial investigation. The patient decided to try a cure with the doctor.

I found a delicate, pale, severely neurasthenic, depressed person, despairing of his future, without external signs of degeneration. The patient recognised his skewed position and seemed to want to do everything in his power to become a proper, decent person again. He deeply lamented his sexual perversion, which he judged to be pathological but acquired. He made no secret of the fact that he was not able to control himself with young men, nor could he stand the thought of having to abstain from masturbation, into which he was forced for lack of something better. Only a powerful will forced upon him could protect him against it.

His male love had hitherto consisted exclusively in mutual masturbation; erection only occurred when he touched a man he loved, ejaculation occurred early, but mere embrace was not enough. He had never felt himself to be in a special sexual role in relation to men, and his genitals and vegetative organs were normal.

In addition to ordering a contra-neurasthenic treatment on 8 April 1890, a hypnotic-suggestive one was started. The hypnosis was easily achieved by mere sight and verbal suggestion. After half a minute, the patient fell into highly diminished sensibility and mobility with cataleptic behaviour of the muscles. The awakening occurred by suggesting awakening while counting to three. Post-hypnotic suggestions were attainable in each case. The intra-hypnotic suggestions extended to

1. *the prohibition of masturbation,*
2. *the command to find male love contemptible, abominable and to declare it impossible,*
3. *the command to find only ladies beautiful, to approach them, to dream of them, to get aroused libido and erection at the sight of them.*

The sessions would take place daily. On 14 April, the patient reported with a kind of moral satisfaction that he had copulated with pleasure and ejaculated tardily.

On the 16th he felt free of masturbatory impulses, attracted to women, completely indifferent to men. He dreams of female charms and female company.

On 1 May, the patient appears and feels sexually quite normal. Psychologically, he has become a completely different personality, full of courage and self-confidence.

He has sex normally with full satisfaction and believes himself safe from relapse.

In a later letter, Mr P. writes:]

As is not otherwise conceivable, I find myself permanently freed from those aberrations. The only thing that still reminds me of the dark time are the rare dreams from the bleak past, which I have no power to banish, and which sometimes even occupy my thoughts in a pleasant way. By my own will, I hope, I will succeed in getting rid of them completely in the near future. Should I ever weaken again, your insistent ideas—I am sure of it—will make me resist vigorously, and I shall not succumb.

[KRAFFT-EBING: On 20 October 1890, P. wrote to me:]

From onanism I am completely cured, and manly love finds no favour with me. However, full potency does not yet seem to have returned, although I live soundly. Nevertheless, I feel satisfied.

Index[1]

[1] Note: Page numbers followed by 'n' refer to notes.

D. Pretsell, *Queer Voices in the Works of Richard von Krafft-Ebing, 1883–1901*, Genders and Sexualities in History,
https://doi.org/10.1007/978-3-031-17331-8

MIX
Papier | Fördert
gute Waldnutzung
FSC® C083411

Kolibri 360 GmbH
Ferdinand-Jühlke-Straße 7
99095 Erfurt, Deutschland
produktsicherheit@kolibri360.de